HIKE LIST

MENASHA RIDGE PRESS
Birmingham, Alabama

60 HIKES WITHIN 60 MILES

SAN ANTONIO
and AUSTIN

INCLUDING
THE HILL COUNTRY

THIRD EDITION

JOHNNY MOLLOY
WITH **TOM TAYLOR**

60 Hikes within 60 Miles: San Antonio & Austin

Copyright © 2010 Johnny Molloy and Tom Taylor
All rights reserved
Printed in the United States of America
Published by Menasha Ridge Press
Distributed by Publishers Group West
Third edition, third printing 2015

Library of Congress Cataloging-in-Publication Data

Molloy, Johnny, 1961-
   60 hikes within 60 miles, San antonio & austin including the hill country / Johnny
   Molloy with Tom Taylor. — 3rd ed.
      p. cm.
   Includes index.
   ISBN-13: 978-0-89732-904-0
   ISBN-10: 0-89732-904-X
   1. Hiking—Texas—San Antonio Region—Guidebooks. 2. Hiking—Texas—Austin
   Region—Guidebooks. 3. Trails—Texas—San Antonio Region—Guidebooks. 4. Trails—
   Texas—Austin Region—Guidebooks. 5. San Antonio Region (Tex.)—Guidebooks. 6.
   Austin Region (Tex.)—Guidebooks. I. Taylor, Tom, 1970- II. Title. III. Title: Sixty
   hikes within sixty miles, San antonio & austin including the hill country.
   GV199.42.T492S366 2010
   796.5109764'3—dc22

                              2010026623

Cover and text design by Steveco International
Cover photo copyright © David Sucsy
   Austin skyline; Congress Avenue Bridge;
   Town Lake; tree-framed cityscape
All other photos by Johnny Molloy
Maps by Steve Jones and Scott McGrew

Menasha Ridge Press
P.O. Box 43673
Birmingham, AL 35243
menasharidge.com

DISCLAIMER

This book is meant only as a guide to select trails in the San Antonio and Austin areas and does not guarantee hiker safety in any way—you hike at your own risk. Neither Menasha Ridge Press, Johnny Molloy, nor Tom Taylor is liable for property loss or damage, personal injury, or death that result in any way from accessing or hiking the trails described in the following pages. Please be aware that hikers have been injured in the San Antonio and Austin areas. Be especially cautious when walking on or near boulders, steep inclines, and drop-offs, and do not attempt to explore terrain that may be beyond your abilities. To help ensure an uneventful hike, please read carefully the introduction to this book, and perhaps get further safety information and guidance from other sources. Familiarize yourself thoroughly with the areas you intend to visit before venturing out. Ask questions, and prepare for the unforeseen. Familiarize yourself with current weather reports, maps of the area you intend to visit, and any relevant park regulations.

FOR ALL THE HIKERS IN THE LONE STAR STATE. — JOHNNY MOLLOY

FOR MY WIFE AND TRAIL PARTNER, DALE. —TOM TAYLOR

TABLE OF CONTENTS

FOREWORD

Welcome to Menasha Ridge Press's *60 Hikes within 60 Miles*. Our strategy was simple: First, find a hiker who knows the area and loves to hike. Second, ask that person to spend a year researching the most popular and very best trails around. And third, have that person describe each trail in terms of difficulty, scenery, condition, elevation change, and all other categories of information that are important to hikers. "Pretend you've just completed a hike and met up with other hikers at the trailhead," we told each author. "Imagine their questions, and be clear in your answers." Experienced hikers and writers, authors Johnny Molloy and Tom Taylor have selected 60 of the best hikes in and around the San Antonio and Austin areas. This third edition includes new hikes. From urban hikes that make use of parklands to aerobic outings in national forests, Molloy and Taylor provide hikers (and walkers) with a great variety of hikes—and all within roughly 60 miles of San Antonio and Austin.

You'll get more out of this book if you take a moment to read the Introduction explaining how to read the trail listings. The Topographic Maps section will help you understand how useful topos will be on a hike and will also tell you where to get them. And though this is a "where-to" rather than a "how-to" guide, those of you who have hiked extensively will find the Introduction of particular value. As much for the opportunity to free the spirit, as well as to free the body, let these hikes elevate you above the urban hurry.

All the best,
The Editors at Menasha Ridge Press

ABOUT THE AUTHORS

JOHNNY MOLLOY is an outdoor writer based in Johnson City, Tennessee. Born in Memphis, he moved to Knoxville in 1980 to attend the University of Tennessee. During his college years, he developed a love of the natural world that has become the primary focus of his life.

It all started on a backpacking foray into Great Smoky Mountains National Park. That first trip was a disaster; nevertheless, Molloy discovered a love of the outdoors that would lead him to canoe-camp and backpack throughout the United States and abroad over the next 25 years. Today, he averages 150 nights out per year.

After graduating from UT in 1987 with a degree in economics, Molloy spent an ever-increasing amount of time in the wild, becoming more skilled in a variety of environments. Friends enjoyed his adventure stories; one even suggested he write a book. He pursued that idea and soon parlayed his love of the outdoors into an occupation.

The results of his efforts are more than 38 books, including hiking, camping, paddling, and other comprehensive guidebooks, as well as books on true outdoor adventures. He has also written numerous articles for magazines and Web sites, and he continues to write and travel extensively to all four corners of the United States, endeavoring in a variety of outdoor pursuits. For the latest on Molloy, visit his Web site, **johnnymolloy.com**.

Whether tracking game, looking for a secluded fishing spot, or just wandering the countryside, **TOM TAYLOR** spends a great deal of time on Texas's trails. A native raised in west Texas, he migrated to the Hill Country area to take advantage of all it has to offer in outdoor recreation. Taylor now resides in San Antonio.

PREFACE

I'm not one who walks for the sake of walking. Exercise isn't a good enough excuse. However, I'll walk for miles to see something that's out of the ordinary or extremely beautiful. I also love to hike just to get away from it all. I think the hikes in this book reflect this. My hope is that you'll enjoy these hikes and find them to be just as interesting as I did.

There are many scenic sights on these trails, from crystalline springs to historic homesteads to waves of Texas Hill Country expanding to the horizon. Sometimes, just the opportunity to see something interesting is enough. The blinds overlooking the Colorado River at Hornsby Bend offer the possibility of some great bird viewing. At the right time of year, you could sit all day in the cool fall air and watch the migrating ducks as they make their way through the central flyway. This is worth the trip, and it's a healthy hike to boot. It's not too challenging and definitely not what you'd expect to find near a water treatment facility. Yet there it is. Interesting.

Following the Twin Peaks hike to its apex will give you the best chance in this part of the country of seeing a mountain lion. They are out there, but you'll have to sit still to catch one in the distance. This won't be a problem, though, because by the time you reach the peak, you'll be ready to rest. Just keep your eyes open.

All of the trails, even ones in the middle of San Antonio or Austin, contain a wide variety of wildlife. McAllister Park, one of the busiest, has one of the largest deer populations of any of the hikes in this book. It's also where I saw the most snakes. If you look hard enough, and are quiet enough, you could see deer at every park and preserve in this book. You'll also find abundant and diverse species of birds.

Texas hosts more than 600 species of birds. Being located in the South Central part of the state, near the woods and the coast, allows you to see a lot of them right here. Rare painted buntings are at McKinney Falls on the Homestead Trail; a large variety of sparrows and finches are everywhere; and cardinals, jays, titmice, and more can be seen on these trails. I've spotted a pileated woodpecker in Buescher State Park. Very rare for these parts. To enrich your bird-watching, pick up a bird guide before you go hiking. I never leave home without my binoculars and bird guide.

Keep your eyes on the ground and you could see everything from coral snakes to the rare Houston toad. Big tarantulas (especially in Buescher) live deeper in the woods too. One of the most fascinating trails for local wildlife is in Lockhart State Park. Huge garden spiders build webs more than 10 feet wide across the trails. You can't miss them, so don't walk into them. Although toads and spiders are creepy to some, these kinds of encounters are worth the drive for me.

Over time some trails change. Some parks close and others open. For example, Commons Ford Ranch was sold and is now in private hands. Yet other places have opened. Government Canyon State Natural Area, just west of San Antonio, offers 8,000 acres to explore via 20-plus miles of hiking trails. Medina River Natural Area has opened. Hikers can travel the river bottoms and see giant ancient cypress and cottonwoods. Other places, such as Palmetto State Park, have revamped their trail systems, bringing about new experiences at old destinations. Guadalupe River State Park expanded its trail network. With this book in hand, you can enjoy the new hikes that include the above areas.

Many hikers in the area make regular use of our extensive range of trails and tend to take good care of them too. Some of the most beautiful trails, and some that would seem more out of the way, see a lot of traffic on weekends. For a better chance at solitude, any of your trips would benefit from going during the week rather than the weekend.

However, at some parks crowding doesn't seem to be related to the time of day or year. McAllister Park is always busy. All day, every day, all year long. The Hill Country SNA sees an awful lot of traffic for its remote location as well. If you're looking for a rugged hike, it's your place, but if you're looking for solitude, it might not be for you. This leads me to my favorite hike of all those in the book . . . .

Friedrich Wilderness Park. This trail is located close to San Antonio and is unique among most trails in our area. It offers a lot of elevation change and seems to have more in common with the mountain states than with Texas. It is very secluded and sees little use. After you've hiked—and climbed—to the stone fence halfway through and realize that you haven't seen anyone else, it'll set in. Just sit on the fence and listen to the silence. It's a great trail, my personal favorite.

All of the parks and trails, however, are worth visiting and, more so, worth preserving. If you get a chance to contribute to a donation box for maintenance, please do so, especially if you enjoyed the trail. Every trail in this book is worth a few dollars to visit.

—*Johnny Molloy, September 2010*

HIKING RECOMMENDATIONS

HIKES 1–3 MILES

HIKES 3–6 MILES

HIKES MORE THAN 6 MILES

HIKES GOOD FOR YOUNG CHILDREN

SCENIC HIKES (continued)

HISTORIC HIKES

HIKES FOR WILDLIFE VIEWING

LESS-BUSY HIKES (continued)

HEAVILY TRAVELED HIKES

INTRODUCTION

Welcome to the third edition of *60 Hikes within 60 Miles: San Antonio and Austin*! If you're new to hiking or even if you're a seasoned trailsmith, take a few minutes to read the following introduction. We explain how this **book** is organized and how to use it.

HIKE DESCRIPTIONS

Each hike contains six key items: a brief description of the trail, a key at-a-glance information box, directions to the trail, a trail map, an elevation profile, and a more detailed trail description, and many hikes also include information about nearby activities. Combined, the maps and information provide a clear method to assess each trail from the comfort of your favorite reading chair.

IN BRIEF

A taste of the trail. Think of this section as a snapshot focused on the historical landmarks, beautiful vistas, and other sights that you may encounter on the trail.

KEY AT-A-GLANCE INFORMATION

The At-a-Glance boxes give you a quick idea of the specifics of each hike. Fourteen basic elements are covered:

LENGTH The length of the trail from start to finish. There may be options to shorten or extend the hikes, but the mileage corresponds to the described hike. Consult the hike description to help decide how to customize the hike for your ability or time constraints.

CONFIGURATION A description of what the trail might look like from overhead. Trails can be loops, out-and-backs (trails on which one enters and leaves along the same path), figure eights, or balloons (trails on which one enters and leaves on

1

the same path with a loop in between). The descriptions might surprise you.

DIFFICULTY The degree of effort an "average" hiker should expect on a given hike. For simplicity, difficulty is described as "easy," "moderate," or "difficult."

SCENERY A rating of the overall environs of the hike and what to expect in terms of plant life, wildlife, streams, and historic buildings.

EXPOSURE A quick check of how much sun you can expect during the hike. Descriptors used include terms such as "shady," "exposed," and "sunny."

TRAFFIC Indicators of how busy the trail might be on an average day, and if you might be able to find solitude out there. Trail traffic, of course, varies from day to day and season to season.

TRAIL SURFACE A description of the trail surface, be it paved, rocky, dirt, or a mixture of elements.

HIKING TIME The length of time it takes to hike the trail. A slow but steady hiker will average 2 to 3 miles an hour, depending on the terrain. Most of the estimates in this book reflect a speed of about 2 miles per hour. Take the miles of the hike and divide by two and this will give a rough estimate of hiking time. For example, an 8-mile hike should take the average hiker 4 hours.

DRIVING DISTANCE This is how far to drive from a given point, in this case, from the state capitol in Austin or the Alamodome in San Antonio.

ACCESS A notation of fees or permits needed to access the trail (if any) and whether the trail has specific hours.

WHEELCHAIR ACCESSIBILITY Notes whether the trail is wheelchair compatible.

MAPS Which map is the best for this hike and where to get it.

FACILITIES What to expect in terms of restrooms, water, and other amenities available at the trailhead or nearby.

CONTACT INFORMATION Gives you contact information, including phone number and Web site, in case you want to do additional research.

DIRECTIONS TO THE TRAIL

The detailed directions will lead you to each trailhead. If you use GPS technology, provided latitude and longitude coordinates allow you to navigate directly to the trailhead.

TRAIL DESCRIPTIONS

The trail description is the heart of each hike. Here, the author provides a summary of the trail's essence and highlights any special traits that the hike offers. Ultimately, the hike description will help you choose which hikes are best for you.

NEARBY ACTIVITIES

Not every hike will have this listing. For those that do, look here for information on nearby dining opportunities or other activities to fill out your day.

MAPS

The maps in this book have been produced with great care and, used with the hiking directions, will help you stay on course. But as any experienced hiker knows, things can get tricky off the beaten path.

The maps in this book, when used with the route directions present in each chapter, are sufficient to direct you to the trail and guide you on it. However, you will find superior detail and valuable information in the United States Geological Survey's 7.5-minute series topographic maps. Topo maps are available online in many locations. The easiest single Web resource is located at **msrmaps.com.** You can view and print topos of the entire Unites States there and view aerial photographs of the same areas. The downside to topos is that most are outdated, having been created 20–30 years ago. But they still provide excellent topographic detail.

If you're new to hiking, you might be wondering, "What's a topographic map?" In short, a topo indicates not only linear distance but elevation as well, using contour lines. Wavy contour lines spread across topo maps, each line representing a particular elevation. At the base of each topo, a contour's interval designation is given. If the contour interval is 200 feet, then the distance between each contour line is 200 feet. Follow five contour lines up on a map and the elevation has increased by 1,000 feet.

Let's assume that the 7.5-minute series topo reads "contour interval 40 feet," that the short trail we'll be hiking is two inches in length on the map, and that it crosses five contour lines from beginning to end. What do we know? Well, because the linear scale of this series is 2,000 feet to the inch (roughly two and three-quarters inches representing 1 mile), we know our trail is approximately four-fifths of a mile long (2 inches are 4,000 feet). But we also know that we'll be climbing or descending 200 vertical feet (5 contour lines are 40 feet each) over that distance. And the elevation designations written on occasional contour lines will tell us if we're heading up or down.

In addition to outdoor shops and bike shops, you'll find topos at major universities and some public libraries, where you might try photocopying the ones you need to avoid the cost of buying them. But if you want your own and can't find them locally, visit the United States Geological Survey Web site at **topo maps.usgs.gov.** I also recommend **topozone.com** and others mentioned in the appendix as resources for topographic maps and software.

THE OVERVIEW MAP AND KEY

Use the overview map on the inside front cover to find the exact location of each hike's primary trailhead. Each hike's number appears on the overview map, on the hike list facing the overview map, and in the table of contents. As you flip through the book, you'll see that a hike's full profile is easy to locate by watching for the hike number at the top of each page. The book is organized by region, as indicated in the table of contents. A map legend that details the symbols found on trail maps appears on the inside back cover.

REGIONAL MAPS

The book is divided into regions, and prefacing each regional section is an overview map of that region. The regional map provides more detail than the overview map does, bringing you closer to the hike.

TRAIL MAPS

Each hike contains a detailed map that shows the trailhead, route, significant features, facilities, and topographic landmarks such as creeks, overlooks, and peaks. The author gathered map data by carrying Garmin eTrex or Garmin 60CS GPS units while hiking. This data was downloaded into the digital mapping program Topo USA and processed by expert cartographers to produce the highly accurate maps found in this book. Each trailhead's GPS coordinates are included with each profile (see below).

ELEVATION PROFILES

Each hike contains a detailed elevation profile that corresponds directly to the trail map. The elevation profile provides a quick look at the trail from the side, enabling you to visualize how it rises and falls. Note the number of feet between each tick mark on the vertical axis (the height scale). To avoid making flat hikes look steep and steep hikes appear flat, height scales are used throughout the book to provide an accurate assessment of each hike's climbing difficulty.

GPS TRAILHEAD COORDINATES

In addition to highly specific trail outlines, this book also includes the latitude/longitude coordinates for each trailhead. The latitude and longitude grid system is likely quite familiar to you, but here is a refresher.

Imaginary lines of latitude—called parallels and approximately 69 miles apart from each other—run horizontally around the globe. Each parallel is indicated by degrees from the equator (established to be 0°): up to 90°N at the North Pole and down to 90°S at the South Pole.

Imaginary lines of longitude—called meridians—run perpendicular to latitude lines. Longitude lines are likewise indicated by degrees: Starting from 0° at the Prime Meridian, in Greenwich, England, they continue to the east and west until they meet 180° later at the International Date Line in the Pacific Ocean. At the equator, longitude lines also are approximately 69 miles apart, but that distance narrows as the meridians converge toward the North and South poles.

Each degree can be divided into 60 minutes and each minute into 60 seconds. This system provides a precise location by the coordinates of the latitude and longitude lines.

For more on GPS technology, the USGS offers a good deal of information regarding UTM coordinates at its Web site, **usgs.gov.**

WEATHER

With the exception of July, August, and September, the weather for hiking in the Hill Country can be great. Even the summer months have cool mornings of which you can take advantage. The best times are October and November and March through May. Depending on the severity of winter, December can be just as pleasant as early fall. The main things to watch out for are the heat, which can be brutal in the summer, and the rains. With all the rivers in the area, flash floods can be a real problem for unwary hikers. The Guadalupe River, for example, has flooded to the point of washing homes away twice in less than 10 years, and it doesn't take long for the waters to reach dangerous levels. What might seem like a pleasant light rain for a hike could turn to disaster. With the heat, hydration is key. Carry lots of water, and get off the trails before morning is gone.

DAILY AVERAGE DAILY TEMPERATURES BY MONTH

	JAN	FEB	MAR	APR	MAY	JUN
HIGH	59° F	63° F	72° F	79° F	85° F	91° F
LOW	39° F	42° F	51° F	60° F	67° F	71° F
	JUL	**AUG**	**SEP**	**OCT**	**NOV**	**DEC**
HIGH	95° F	96° F	90° F	82° F	72° F	62° F
LOW	74° F	74° F	70° F	60° F	50° F	41° F

TRAIL ETIQUETTE

Whether you're on a city, county, state, or national park trail, always remember that great care and resources (from nature as well as from your tax dollars) have gone into creating these trails. Treat the trail, wildlife, and fellow hikers with respect.

1. **Hike on open trails only. Respect trail and road closures (ask if not sure), avoid possible trespassing on private land, and obtain permits and authorization as required. Leave gates as you found them or as marked.**

2. **Leave only footprints. Be sensitive to the ground beneath you. This also means staying on the trail and not creating any new ones. Be sure to pack out what you pack in. No one likes to see the trash someone else has left behind.**

3. **Never spook animals. An unannounced approach, a sudden movement, or a loud noise startles all animals. This can be dangerous for you, for others, and for the animals. Give animals extra room and time to adjust to you.**

4. **Plan ahead. Know your equipment, your ability, and the area in which you are hiking—and prepare accordingly. Be self-sufficient at all times; carry**

necessary supplies for changes in weather or other conditions. A well-executed trip is a satisfaction to you and to others.

5. Be courteous to other hikers, bikers, or equestrians you meet on the trails.

WATER

"How much is enough? One bottle? Two? Three? But think of all that extra weight!" Well, one simple physiological fact should convince you to err on the side of excess when it comes to deciding how much water to pack: a hiker working hard in 90° heat needs approximately 10 quarts of fluid every day. That's two and a half gallons—12 large water bottles or 16 small ones. In other words, pack along one or two bottles even for short hikes.

Serious backpackers hit the trail prepared to purify water found along the route. This method, while less dangerous than drinking it untreated, comes with risks. Purifiers with ceramic filters are the safest but are also the most expensive. Many hikers pack along the slightly distasteful tetraglycine hydroperiodide tablets (sold under the names Potable Aqua, Coughlan's, and others).

If you're tempted to drink "found" water, do so only if you understand the risks involved. Probably the most common water-borne "bug" that hikers face is *giardia,* which may not hit until one to four weeks after ingestion. It will have you passing noxious rotten-egg gas, vomiting, shivering with chills, and living in the bathroom. But there are other parasites to worry about, including E. coli and cryptosporidium (that are harder to kill than *giardia*).

For most people, the pleasures of hiking make carrying water a relatively minor price to pay to remain healthy. If you're tempted to drink "found water," do so only if you understand the risks involved. Better yet, hydrate prior to your hike, carry (and drink) six ounces of water for every mile you plan to hike, and hydrate after the hike.

FIRST-AID KIT

A typical kit may contain more items than you might think necessary. But these are just the basics. Pack the items in a waterproof bag, such as a plastic zip-top bag or a similar product.

Ace bandages or Spenco joint wraps

Antibiotic ointment (Neosporin or the generic equivalent)

Aspirin, ibuprofen, or acetaminophen

Band-Aids

Benadryl or the generic equivalent, diphenhydramine (in case of allergic reactions)

Butterfly-closure bandages

Epinephrine in a prefilled syringe (for people known to have severe allergic reactions to such things as bee stings)

Gauze and compress pads (one roll and a half-dozen 4- x 4-inch pads)

Hydrogen peroxide, Betadine, or iodine

Matches or pocket lighter

Moleskin

Sunscreen

Water purification tablets or water filter (see "Water" on page 6)

Whistle (it's more effective in signaling rescuers than your voice)

HIKING WITH CHILDREN

No one is ever too young for a nice hike in the woods or through a city park. Parents with infants can strap on little ones with the popular Snugli device. Be careful, though. Flat, short trails are probably best with an infant. Toddlers who have not quite mastered walking can still tag along, riding on an adult's back in a child carrier.

Children who are walking can, of course, follow along with an adult. Use common sense to judge a child's capacity to hike a particular trail. Always rely on the possibility that the child will tire quickly and have to be carried.

When packing for the hike, remember the needs of the child as well as your own. Make sure children are adequately clothed for the weather, have proper shoes, and are properly protected from the sun with sunscreen and clothing. Kids can dehydrate quickly, so make sure you have plenty of fluid for everyone.

Depending on age, ability, and the hike's length and difficulty, most children should enjoy the shorter hikes described in this book. To assist an adult with determining which trails are suitable for children, a list of hike recommendations for children is provided on pages XII–XIII.

THE BUSINESS HIKER

Whether in the San Antonio–Austin area on business, as a resident, or as a visitor, you'll find many quick getaways perfect for a long lunch escape or an evening hike to unwind from a busy day at the office or convention. Instead of staying cooped up inside, head out to one of the many parks and conservation areas on the fringes of the metro area and combine lunch with a relaxing walk.

TICKS

Ticks like to hang out in the brush that grows along trails. July is a peak month for ticks, but you should be tick-aware during all months of the spring, summer, and fall. Ticks, actually arthropods and not insects, are ectoparasites, which need a host for the majority of their life cycle in order to reproduce. The ticks that light onto you while hiking will be very small, sometimes so tiny that you won't be able to spot them. Primarily of two varieties, deer ticks and dog ticks, both need a few hours of actual attachment before they can transmit any disease they may harbor. I've found ticks in my socks and on my legs several hours after a hike that have not yet anchored. The best strategy is to visually check every half hour or so while hiking, do a thorough check before you get in the car, and then, when you take a posthike shower, do an even more thorough check of your entire body. Ticks that haven't latched on are easily removed but not easily killed. If I pick off a tick in the woods, I just toss it aside. If I find one on my person at home, I make sure to dispatch it down the toilet. For ticks that have embedded, removal with tweezers is best.

POISON IVY, OAK, AND SUMAC

Recognizing and avoiding contact with poison ivy, oak, and sumac is the most effective way to prevent the painful, itchy rashes associated with these plants. Poison ivy occurs as a vine or shrub, with 3 leaflets to a leaf; poison oak occurs as either a vine or shrub, with 3 leaflets as well; and poison sumac flourishes in swampland, with each leaf containing 7 to 13 leaflets. Urushiol, the oil in the sap of these plants, is responsible for the rash.

Within 12–24 hours of exposure, raised lines and/or blisters will appear, accompanied by a terrible itch. Refrain from scratching because bacteria under fingernails may cause infection. Wash and dry the rash thoroughly, applying a calamine lotion to help dry out the rash. If itching or blistering is severe, seek medical attention. If you do come into contact with one of these plants, remember that oil-contaminated clothes, pets, or hiking gear can easily inflict an irritating rash on you or someone else, so wash not only any exposed parts of your body but also clothes, gear, and pets, if applicable.

Austin (Hikes 1-18)

N

0   4.5   9
miles

Liberty Hill
San Gabriel River
Lake Georgetown
Georgetown
San Gabriel River
29
183
29
130
Round Mountain
Rabbit Hill
183A
FM 1431
35
79
Brushy Creek
Round Mountain Road
Cedar Park
Round Rock
45
8
FM 718
Wells Branch
130
FM 973
Lake Travis
Comanche Peak
13
183
1
17
15
360
2
275
290
Colorado Creek
5
35
Walter E. Long Lake
Bee Cave
18
1
11
AUSTIN
130
FM 969
Barton Creek
14
16
71
10
183
71
Oak Hill
360
275
4
Del Valle
Colorado River
12
3
71
Garfield
Signal Hill
7
6 9
290
Dee Gabriel Collins Road
Buda
21
FM 1321
Cedar Creek
35
183
Onion Creek
Mendoza
Blanco Creek
21

AUSTIN

01 BARTON CREEK GREENBELT

KEY AT-A-GLANCE INFORMATION

LENGTH: 8.5 miles

CONFIGURATION: Out-and-back

DIFFICULTY: Difficult

SCENERY: River canyon, riparian woods, clear stream

EXPOSURE: Mostly shady

TRAFFIC: Heavy

TRAIL SURFACE: Dirt, rocks

HIKING TIME: 5.5 hours

DRIVING DISTANCE: 3 miles from the state capitol

ACCESS: Daily, 5 a.m.–10 p.m.; no fees or permits

WHEELCHAIR ACCESS: No

MAPS: ci.austin.tx.us/parks/ parkdirectory.htm

FACILITIES: Restrooms, water at trailhead; restroom also along trail

CONTACT INFORMATION: (512) 476-9044; ci.austin.tx.us/parks

GPS TRAILHEAD COORDINATES

LATITUDE: 30° 26' 50.00"
LONGITUDE: 97° 76' 67.50"

IN BRIEF

This out-and-back hike travels up the canyon of Barton Creek from Barton Springs Pool at Zilker Park to the MoPac Bridge near Twin Falls. Along the way, you will see rock bluffs overlooking a clear blue stream bordered by riparian hardwood forests as well as drier woods of cedar. The crystalline stream not only has scenic shoals but also deep pools for swimming and stone bluffs popular with rock climbers.

DESCRIPTION

This is, in my humble opinion, one of the best urban hikes in America. Barton Creek Greenbelt is an oasis of nature in the middle of central Austin. While here, you can enjoy a clear stream that has cut a canyon over time, showing off its geologic history in the sheer walls that accompany the stream most of the way. Rich vegetation accompanies the rocks and stream in the form of streamside trees such as sycamore and elm. In other places live oak and cedar grow. The entire picture adds up to a

----

Directions ⟶

From I-35 in downtown Austin, take Exit 233, Town Lake/Riverside Drive. Cross Town Lake to reach Riverside Drive. Head west on Riverside Drive and follow it 1.1 miles to Barton Springs Road. Turn left on Barton Springs Road and follow it 1.3 miles to Zilker Park. Turn left again on Barton Springs Road (a park road) and follow it to end in a parking lot just past the Barton Springs Pool entrance. The Barton Creek Greenbelt starts at the west end of the parking area. The safest parking is directly in front of the pool entrance area. Be aware that this trail sometimes closes after rainy periods. If you are in doubt, call ahead; (512) 472-1267.

N

0   0.2   0.4

mile

Barton Springs Pool Building

Barton Springs Rd.

Town Lake

Barton Springs Pool

Zilker Path

P

Spyglass Access

Barton Creek

Gus Fruh Access

Three Falls

MoPac

Loop 360 Access

Frontage Road

MoPac

Frontage Road

cliff face with chain handhold

Loop 360/Capital of TX Hwy.

Twin Falls-Gaines Access

Twin Falls

MoPac

(Trail is on both sides of creek west of MoPac.)

FEET

700
650
600
550
500
450
400
350
300

2   4   6   8   8.5

MILES

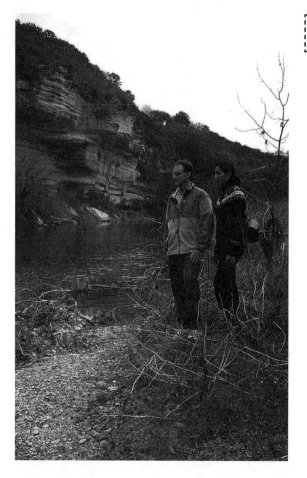

Admiring the canyon stream

wilderness feel, about as wild as you are going to get with skyscrapers and interstates nearby. You will hear the sounds of civilization in the distance, but in other places you'll hear nothing but flowing water cascading over rocks, continuing to carve and shape this preserve.

Leave the trailhead and begin heading upstream on a gravel path. Barton Creek is to your left as you pass through a field. Shortly enter the canyon of the stream. The trail is marked in quarter-mile increments. The forest-banked creek, which is littered with whitish boulders, forms riffles and shoals. Gravel bars border much of the clear watercourse, where you can easily view the bottom. Bluffs appear at 0.5 miles. Don't be surprised if you see rock climbers plying the bluffs, helmets on, colorful ropes attached.

In places, the trail splits. One route will be for bikers, the other for hikers. In other places, the main trail splits out from previous hikers taking multiple routes. However, it is hard to get truly lost because the river and the canyon keep you in line.

At 1 mile the Spyglass Access Trail leaves to the right. A little store sells food and drinks at the road access. A restroom is near the junction. Beyond here the canyon widens out and the sky opens overhead. Straddle the divide between the riparian vegetation and the thicker forest.

At 1.5 miles the trail crosses Barton Creek. Depending on the flow, the crossing may be a wet-footed ford. A secondary path stays upstream without crossing, staying along the edge of a bluff. Rock climbers are frequently over there. The primary path borders lower canyon walls. Look left for a fissure in the wall, forming a small cave. The now-narrow path dips and rolls between trees and over rocks.

At 2.5 miles the Gus Fruh Access cuts off to the left. A nice gravel bar and contemplation bench overlook Barton Creek here. This is also the point where the greenbelt crosses over to the right-hand bank as you head upstream. This crossing can be dry over rocks most of the year, but look for deeper swimming holes nearby. Keep upstream in rich woods before the trail returns creekside near a white-walled canyon. More deep pools are here. Then reach the Three Falls: Just as it sounds, three back-to-back cascades descend the canyon.

The main trail crosses over to the far bank of Barton Creek just past Three Falls. Again, a secondary trail stays along the right bank, eliminating the ford. The main trail, on the left bank, traverses a boardwalk spanning a side stream. Here, as in many places, separate hiking and biking trails diverge. The hiking trail generally stays closer to Barton Creek. Just ahead at 3.5 miles is the Loop 360 Access. A rock climbers' bluff is just across the creek from the Loop 360 Access trail. Keep forward to pass under noisy Loop 360, Capital of Texas Highway.

Beyond the bridge the trail drifts away from the creek at times. Many live oaks thrive here. The path narrows, returns to the creek, and begins to hug a bluff line to your left. The bluff narrows so much at one point that a chain has been put into the bluff and footholds have been dug to aid hikers and keep them from falling in the creek. Stay along the bluff line amid some of the greenbelt's best scenery. Overhanging rock, green ferns, and shade make this a desirable spot on a hot day. A deep pool adds to the mix. The valley widens, and the greenbelt reaches a very deep pool with a rope swing tied to a live oak. This makes for a good stopping spot, though the MoPac Bridge is nearby. The MoPac Bridge can be your official turnaround spot. However, if you want to make it a 4.5-mile one-way hike, you can end at the Twin Falls–Gaines Access. But you must cross Barton Creek to reach the Twin Falls–Gaines Access. The official crossing (no bridge) is upstream about a quarter mile near Twin Falls. Then you backtrack a bit to reach the 0.2-mile ascent to the access parking area. However, you can just cross over at any shallow spot shortly after the MoPac Bridge. Then keep upstream to reach the access trail. To leave a car at this upper access, see the directions for the Sculpture Falls Hike on the Barton Creek Greenbelt.

NEARBY ACTIVITIES

Zilker Park, at the trailhead, offers swimming at Barton Springs, the Zilker Zephyr (a mini-train to ride), a picnic area, and a hillside theater.

02 BULL CREEK GREENBELT

KEY AT-A-GLANCE INFORMATION

LENGTH: 4 miles

CONFIGURATION: Out-and-back

DIFFICULTY: Easy

SCENERY: Riparian woodland and water

EXPOSURE: Mostly shady

TRAFFIC: Light

TRAIL SURFACE: Dirt

HIKING TIME: 2.5 hours

DRIVING DISTANCE: 14 miles from the state capitol

ACCESS: Daily, 5 a.m.–10 p.m.; no fees or permits

WHEELCHAIR ACCESS: No

MAPS: ci.austin.tx.us/parks/parkdirectory.htm

FACILITIES: Restrooms at both ends of trail

CONTACT INFORMATION: (512) 974-6700; ci.austin.tx.us/parks

GPS TRAILHEAD COORDINATES

LATITUDE: : 30° 36' 93.06"
LONGITUDE: 97° 78' 56.39"

IN BRIEF

This secluded area of south Austin is conspicuously located right under one of its busiest roads. An array of birds and creek dwellers await informed hikers.

DESCRIPTION

The park in which this hike starts is in a familiar place. A small parking lot, restrooms, and a couple of picnic tables stand silently in this quiet little area. The creek forms a pool suitable for swimming in the park, and remnants of a former dam still stand. Neighborhoods encroach on the area, and numerous homes are visible when you drive up to the park, though they'll soon fade from view on the trail.

Along with the obvious draw of the swimming hole in the warmer months, this park has another advantage. Signs about 20 yards from the creek proclaim that from that point on, dogs are not required to be leashed. Fido is free to run and play in the stream just like everyone else, as long as he behaves.

The actual trail begins on the far (east) side of the creek, and crossing should not be a problem. Even in higher water, outcrops help you stay dry. When the water is rushing, however, err on the side of caution. Even the smallest trickle can become a raging river when the rains come. After crossing the creek, look for the obvious trail to your left. You'll find a clear footpath into the brush and trees.

Directions

From the northern part of Austin, head south on Loop 360 and turn left at Lakewood. Parking is located off Loop 360. From the south, reverse the turn direction.

Not far beyond this, you'll reach an intersection. Turn left here and begin following the creek. Numerous spur trails to your left lead down to the creek; many are no more distinct than a game trail.

After you've hiked 0.5 miles, the foliage to the left opens up to reveal a wonderful view of the creek, about 15 feet below. From this vantage point on the stone escarpment, you can watch the creek's inhabitants, including turtles, fish, and salamanders, depending on where the sun is. The glare will make it a little more difficult to see through the water, so polarized sunglasses may be in order. As you continue hiking toward Loop 360, the creek and trail almost merge as you get ready to pass under the highway. The trail gets extremely narrow as it passes through some very tall grass. Once on the other side, you'll see a brown stake and sign marking the trail. You'll encounter a few more of these markers along the hike.

Once beyond the underpass, the trail widens a little, and the hike is easy from here. Keep an eye on the trees as well as the creek. The abundance of water and cover provide ideal habitat for birds of all types, and cardinals appear to be especially common. The birds dart back and forth across the trail along the entire hike. You'll reach a stone staircase after a mile that leads up to a wrought-iron fence. There is no gate apparent. You'll reach a fork just past this point. Stay to the right.

Roughly 0.2 miles from the fork, you'll cross Spicewood Springs Road and see another park on your left about 30 yards away. Keep going across the road, and cross under Loop 360 again. This is the second creek crossing you'll encounter. Before you cross over the creek and under the overpass, take a moment to look up at the bottom of the road. Several cliff swallows have chosen to build their homes here. The mud nests hang upside down from their base and make for an interesting sight.

You'll cross the creek on several square stones, many of which have been marked by passersby. Here the creek widens as it heads back under Loop 360 and offers a beautiful view. Wading birds like egrets and herons can be seen here in the warmer months and make for a striking contrast to the bustle of the busy highway. From this point, the trail continues north, away to the left of the creek.

At 1.5 miles from the trailhead you'll cross another creek bed for a perennial stream. In the middle of this creek bed stands the most curious thing you'll find on this hike—an old red fire hydrant, undisturbed by anything, and not of any obvious use. Beyond the creek the trail will fork again and is clearly marked by another sign, designating the fork to the right as the hiking trail. Go with the sign and continue to the right. The trail opens up past the fork, and the houses are visible again on your right and the highway on the left. A fence is also here on the right, with a sign designating the other side as a restoration area.

The trail forks again at 2 miles, and the trail to the left leads to the Spicewood Springs Road parking lot. This is the turnaround spot, unless you brought two cars and left one here.

HOMESTEAD TRAIL 03

IN BRIEF

This rugged hike passes through land once owned by Thomas F. McKinney, a frontiersman and entrepreneur who greatly influenced the early history of Texas. Share the path with mountain bikers as it meanders through wooded settings and ends by the remains of the McKinney homestead.

DESCRIPTION

The 744 acres of McKinney Falls State Park were part of a much larger (40,000-acre) tract of land once owned by Thomas F. McKinney, a former Kentuckian who made his living as a trader of cotton and livestock. McKinney, along with Stephen F. Austin and others, helped gain statehood for Texas.

The position of the Texas Parks and Wildlife Department is that McKinney was one of Austin's original colonists, but many other reliable sources suggest that he stopped here in the 1820s only to receive his land grant before moving on to the Galveston area, where he set up a trading business and even worked as a privateer during the Texas Revolution, which he also helped finance to the sum of $99,000. When he did settle in this area between 1850 and 1852 to breed racehorses, he also built one of the first flour mills in the area, powered by the Onion Creek. The ruins of the mill and his house are located on this hike.

Getting to this hike's trailhead is a little tricky. After you've parked your car and made your way to the creek, you'll encounter the

----

Directions ———————————————→

From downtown Austin take US 183 south to McKinney Falls Parkway, which will lead right into the park.

KEY AT-A-GLANCE INFORMATION

LENGTH: 3 miles

CONFIGURATION: Loop

DIFFICULTY: Moderate

SCENERY: Old ruins and thick hardwoods

EXPOSURE: Mostly shady with a few openings

TRAFFIC: Light, but watch for mountain bikers

TRAIL SURFACE: Dirt

HIKING TIME: 1.5 hours

DRIVING DISTANCE: 10 miles from the state capitol

ACCESS: Daily, 8 a.m.–10 p.m.; $5 entrance fee/person over age 13

WHEELCHAIR ACCESS: No

MAPS: Available at park office or at tpwd.state.tx.us/publications

FACILITIES: Restrooms, showers, picnic tables, and camping. Many stores are located nearby.

CONTACT INFORMATION: (512) 243-1643; tpwd.state.tx.us/spdest/findadest/parks/mckinney_falls

GPS TRAILHEAD COORDINATES

LATITUDE: : 30° 18' 64.44"
LONGITUDE: 97° 72' 06.11"

toughest part of this trek—crossing the creek to get to the trailhead. The best way to do this without getting your boots wet is to cross along the waterfall. Depending on the time of year and the recent rainfall, this can be somewhat difficult. The limestone bed of the creek has several rocks that stick up out of the water, and these can function as stepping-stones. This is a good hike to bring a walking staff on, if for no other reason than to balance yourself while crossing the water.

Once you've completed the crossing, an obvious sign marks the beginning of the trail. The Homestead ruins are to the left, and the gristmill's remnants are to the right. Follow the trail toward the gristmill. Mountain bikers tend to start riding the Homestead Trail; hiking the other way (counterclockwise) will give you a chance to see each other and avoid a collision later on down the trail.

The remains of the old gristmill are located less than 200 yards from the trailhead and are marked with an information sign. The stones that made up the mill's foundation are all that remain now, but it once was the first working flour mill in the area. Notice how the creek's path has diverted from the mill since it was originally built.

Just over 0.5 miles into the hike, a concrete picnic table sits to the side of the trail. Not marked on the trail map, this would be a good place to get away from the crowds on an otherwise busy day.

Shortly after the picnic table, the trail narrows to allow for only a single hiker at a time. Many small, seasonal creek beds cross the trail, and many are just as wide as the trail itself. As a general rule, keep going straight at these crossings.

The trail forks 0.8 miles from the beginning. Stay to the left; the right fork dead-ends at an open field. You can hear vehicular traffic from across the field, which will remind you just how close you are to the city.

Once you've passed the field, the trees get thick and the birds become very vocal. This part of the trail is great for locating a couple of hard-to-find species. Painted buntings are abundant in these woods, and the occasional indigo bunting will make the walk extremely popular with birders. Their calls will drown out any traffic along the nearby roads. Keep an eye on the trail ahead to see them crossing.

As the trail begins to cut west, a large opening appears on the right, revealing a large building across an open field of wildflowers, about 0.5 miles from the picnic table. This is part of the Texas Parks and Wildlife (TPW) headquarters building. From this point the trail cuts west and back into the thick woods.

A little farther up the trail, you'll encounter another part of the TPW complex. This building is a fitness center for TPW employees. Stay on the trail, and pass the facility on the left.

As the trail turns north, you'll reach a small wooden bridge spanning an empty creek bed. This is a good place to take a break and have a look down the creek for deer, birds, or other active wildlife. This bridge is located just before the halfway point, and the trail starts to narrow even more from here.

Along the trail from the bridge you'll begin to see small signs with arrows pointing the way you came. These are for the bikers' benefit, to keep them on the trail and out of the bushes. You don't have to turn around and go back.

The wildflowers are abundant and the grass is tall in a few open areas along the trail, but don't be tempted to wander off the trail. A rattlesnake in the field alerted me to his presence, and you don't want to see them any more than they want to see you.

The tree growth along this part of the trail appears older than in the beginning, and this is a great place to see wildlife. Blue jays and cardinals crisscross the trail, and you can hear the buntings' songs (a triple-note tune that stands out from anything else in the area) again. You can also keep an eye to the right for approaching bikers, as the trail loops back a couple of times.

At almost 3 miles into the hike, you'll reach the old McKinney homestead. The ruins have been stabilized to prevent further loss of the historical building. A barbed wire fence surrounds it, so you'll have to appreciate it from a distance. The trail here widens to road size. Look for a small trail to the right. This will take you back to the trailhead and the end of the hike. Once you cross the creek, you might want to stop and soak your feet in it for a while.

HORNSBY BEND LOOP

IN BRIEF

This unusual trail circles a wastewater treatment plant with numerous ponds near the Colorado River. Before you cry foul, realize that this area is a haven for wildlife of all kinds, especially waterfowl and other types of birds.

DESCRIPTION

Talk about turning lemons into lemonade! The Hornsby Bend Biosolids Management Facility performs the unpleasant but necessary job of processing sewage for the city of Austin. Normally outdoor enthusiasts would avoid such a facility. However, this plant near the banks of the Colorado is a bird-watcher's paradise with trails for viewing the winged critters. A nice 3-plus-mile loop explores the river and its attendant flood plain, along with four ponds where hundreds of birds may be seen. Bring your binoculars and bird book and prepare for an eye-opening event. Bobcats, beavers, coyotes, and deer also call the 700-acre facility home. (I saw several deer during my hike.)

On your first visit, the many buildings, fences, and power lines may make you wonder if you are heading the right way or trespassing. Rest assured, the public is welcome. Leave

Directions ⟶

From the Austin airport take TX 71 east for 1 mile to FR 973. Turn left on FR 973, toward Manor, crossing the Colorado River, following it 1 mile to the Hornsby Bend Biosolids Processing Center. Turn left and follow the wide road as it narrows to pass through a metal gate. Stay with the road for 0.7 miles to near the end of the pavement by Building #10. The hike starts on the gated grassy dike beyond the end of the pavement. The northwest corner of Pond 1 West will be near the parking area.

KEY AT-A-GLANCE INFORMATION

LENGTH: 3.3 miles

CONFIGURATION: Loop

DIFFICULTY: Easy

SCENERY: River flood plain, man-made ponds, buildings

EXPOSURE: Mostly open

TRAFFIC: Light

TRAIL SURFACE: Grass, dirt, pavement

HIKING TIME: 2 hours

DRIVING DISTANCE: 7 miles from the state capitol

ACCESS: Daily, sunrise–sunset; no fees or permits

WHEELCHAIR ACCESS: Mostly handicap accessible, with some assistance

MAPS: hornsbybend.org

FACILITIES: Water, restrooms at administrative offices

CONTACT INFORMATION: (512) 972-1960; hornsbybend.org

GPS TRAILHEAD COORDINATES

LATITUDE: : 30° 22' 33.33"
LONGITUDE: 97° 63' 77.78"

0   0.15   0.3

mile

FR 973

To 71
& Austin

composting and
drying basin

Pond 1 East

Black
Willow
Trl.

buildings

Pond 1 West

Pond 2

P

Supper Island
View Trail

Pond 3

Colorado River

River Trail.

71

Bastrop Hwy.

FEET						
700						
650						
600						
550						
500						
450						
400						
350						
300						

0.5   1   1.5   2   2.5   3   3.3

MILES

Bird life is abundant at Hornsby Bend.

your parking spot near the end of Pond 1 West and then keep west across the gated dike with an adjacent power line. This is the River Trail. Pond 3 is to your left and is marshy with grasses and trees—unlike the other ponds, which are mostly open. At 0.3 miles the Colorado River comes into view. A spur trail leads forward to reach the river's edge. This hike, however, turns left along with the dike to continue skirting Pond 3.

You'll reach a greenhouse at 1 mile. Keep behind the building along a paved road that runs between the building and the river; leave the pavement and dip to the bottomland. Ahead, the Upper Island View Trail leads to a view of an island in the Colorado. A primitive viewing blind has been constructed. The river habitat will probably have different birds than those in the treatment ponds. Night herons, cormorants, and kingfishers can be spotted along the Colorado.

Return to the River Trail. Ahead, another spur leads right toward the island. On a curve of the River Trail, the Black Willow Trail also leads to the Colorado. Finally, the River Trail leaves the Colorado and heads toward the ponds, reaching the first one at 2 miles. You are at the southeast corner of Pond 2, the longest pond. A bird blind to your left is a worthwhile side trip. (Hundreds of waterfowl were in the ponds on my visit.) Season, weather, and water-level conditions have everything to do with what you will see. On any given day an experienced birder will observe more than 50 species. To really see the birds, take your time.

The hike keeps north on the paved road to reach a dike between Pond 2 and Pond 1 East. Turn left onto this dirt road, which offers maximum water observation, with ponds all around. Reach the end of the ponds and some outbuildings. Turn right and return to your point of origin.

05 MAYFIELD PRESERVE GARDEN WALK AND AMBLE

KEY AT-A-GLANCE INFORMATION

LENGTH: 1 mile

CONFIGURATION: Multiple interconnected trails

DIFFICULTY: Very easy

SCENERY: Formal gardens, creek gorge, lake

EXPOSURE: Mostly shady

TRAFFIC: Moderate–busy

TRAIL SURFACE: Concrete, dirt, rock

HIKING TIME: 1 hour

DRIVING DISTANCE: 5 miles from the state capitol

ACCESS: Daily, sunrise–sunset; no fees or permits

WHEELCHAIR ACCESS: Yes

MAPS: Signboard map at trailhead

FACILITIES: Picnic area, restroom at trailhead

CONTACT INFORMATION: (512) 974-6700; ci.austin.tx.us/parks

GPS TRAILHEAD COORDINATES

LATITUDE:: 30° 31' 38.61"
LONGITUDE: 97° 76' 91.11"

IN BRIEF

This walk takes place at Mayfield Park Preserve, site of the Mayfield-Gutsch Home and Gardens. After touring the homesite and backyard gardens, amble around on a series of short, interconnected trails through the woods along Bull Creek near the shores of Lake Austin.

DESCRIPTION

To call something a hike implies using a determined trail or set of trails in a specific order, heading from point A to point B. Most hikes will also lead you back from point B to point A. Here at Mayfield Nature Preserve, point A is the parking area, and your starting point is set. The problem is getting to point B and exploring the highlights of this area. Mayfield Nature Preserve has many highlights: the Mayfield-Gutsch House and Gardens, Bull Creek and its canyon scenery, a couple of overhanging rock houses, thick woods, and a vantage point overlooking Lake Austin. The problem is the seemingly innumerable short trails that crisscross this preserve. There is simply no way to systematically walk them to see everything. So just get out here and get lost!

There is no way to be truly lost for more than a few minutes because the park is bounded on all sides by houses, 35th Street, and Lake Austin. In fact, it is a good place to just amble around and let your feet take you where they may, even if it is to a dead end or a backtrack.

Directions

From MoPac, Loop Road 1 in Austin, take 35th Street west for 0.6 miles and prepare to veer left just past Balcones Street, staying on 35th Street for 0.2 miles farther. Turn left into the small stone-gated entrance on your left.

N

0   150   300

feet

To MoPac & Austin

Bull Creek

rock house

rock house

West 35th St.

Mayfield-Gutsch House

stone fence

P

Bull Creek

FEET

700
650
600
550
500
450
400
350
300

0.25   0.5   0.75   1

MILES

Mayfield-Gutsch House

Step back 100 years and learn how Mayfield Park came to be. Alison May-field, Texas Secretary of State from 1894 to 1896 and then Railroad Commis-sioner from 1896 to 1922, purchased the property in 1909. A small cottage was already here, dating from the 1870s. Mayfield used this getaway primarily as a summer cottage. She bequeathed it to her daughter Mary and son-in-law Milton Gutsch in 1922. Milton and Mary began to develop gardens around the house and kept at it for nearly 50 years, building ponds, stone walls, and outbuildings. The house was enlarged as well, ending up as a sprawling cottage. In 1971 the property was bequeathed to the city of Austin for use as a park. In 1994 the park was listed on the National Register of Historic Places. Today you can tour the gardens in addition to walking the mini-maze of trails. The house can be rented for special functions as well.

The following is a suggestion for exploring Mayfield Nature Preserve. Do not worry about following this route directly, for you will get lost, backtrack, and return to the house and parking area a few times, just as I did. Remember that this is an amble, not a true hike, so just let your feet lead the way.

Leave the parking area and take the visitors' entrance to the house and gar-dens. An iron gate allows passage beyond the stone wall. Pass by the front of the house, noting the native Texas palms, which lend a tropical look. Head down the driveway around to the back of the house. Four concrete ponds lie around a smaller center pond, and benches overlook the ponds. Various small gardens, tended by volunteers, grow between the ponds and the back stone wall. Stroll among the gardens, seeing the varied plant species. Look over the back wall of the backyard. The stone wall is backed against the edge of the canyon wall of Bull Creek, which flows below. You will undoubtedly notice the peacocks roaming about the backyard as well.

After you've finished touring the gardens, look for the stone gate with a bell hanging just beneath a stone arbor near the driveway. Enter the woods beyond the gate. The contrast with the landscaped gardens is startling. Nature grows in organic shapes, sizes, and locations. Cedars and live oaks stand tall over their fallen leaves. The path immediately drops down to a feeder branch of Bull Creek. Walk down the creek and rock-hop over it. Look up at the sheer canyon wall. Do you see the back wall of the Mayfield House gardens? Shortly cross Bull Creek, or you could head upstream on the creek.

The multitude of paths soon becomes evident. All the paths are short, so you can get lost and quickly backtrack—or end up having even more fun. Head left past Bull Creek, and you will come to a trail that leads left to a canyon wall. Cedar steps lead up to a couple of small rock houses. (I imagined someone huddling under the shelter during a thunderstorm.)

Now start working toward Lake Austin. The dense woods and numerous trails add a confusing aspect to the walk. Remember that Bull Creek leads to the lake. Spur trails end at the water's edge, where you can overlook Lake Austin. One spur leads to a short boardwalk. You can look into the Bull Creek embayment and the houses across the water. A lucky ambler will keep curving around the edge of the preserve and end up at the parking area. Fear not, for 35th Street and the lake will force you back to the parking area. Once at the parking area, consider another look at the gardens and make another amble of this special swath of Austin.

NEARBY ACTIVITIES

Tour the Austin Museum of Art next door while you are in the area. For more information visit **amoa.org**. *Note:* The Mayfield-Gutsch House and Gardens can be rented for special events.

06 MCKINNEY ROUGHS BOTTOMS AND BLUFFS HIKE

KEY AT-A-GLANCE INFORMATION

LENGTH: 5.7 miles

CONFIGURATION: Figure eight

DIFFICULTY: Moderate–difficult

SCENERY: River vistas, woods, river bottoms

EXPOSURE: Half sunny, half shady

TRAFFIC: Moderate

TRAIL SURFACE: Pea gravel, rocks, dirt

HIKING TIME: 3 hours

DRIVING DISTANCE: 24 miles from the state capitol

ACCESS: Monday–Saturday, 8 a.m.–5 p.m.; Sunday, noon–5 p.m.; $4 entrance fee/person over age 13

WHEELCHAIR ACCESS: Yes, first 0.5 miles of hike

MAPS: lcra.org/library/media/public/docs/community/community_mck_roughs_trailmap.pdf

FACILITIES: Picnic area, restroom at park office

CONTACT INFORMATION: (512) 303-5073; lcra.org/parks/developed_parks/mckinney_roughs.html

GPS TRAILHEAD COORDINATES

LATITUDE:: 30° 14' 26.94"
LONGITUDE: 97° 45' 72.22"

IN BRIEF

This figure-eight loop hike offers views from up high and big trees from down low. Start along the rim of the Colorado River to enjoy some far-reaching vistas. More vantage points can be had on riverside hills. Then dip down to water level, traversing some rich bottomland where massive pecan trees grow. A few last views await on your return to the plateau rim.

DESCRIPTION

McKinney Roughs Nature Park has numerous short trails, and this hike has many trail intersections. However, the trail junctions are well marked, so don't get bogged down in trying to figure out where you are. This loop offers much to see, and the many paths take you to some of the best of the Roughs—views of the Colorado River Valley, through rich forests, directly along the Colorado River, and among bottomland where pecan trees grow to staggering sizes. So study the paths and then take off on an enjoyable trek. Note that the hike travels both hiker and hiker/equestrian trails.

Leave the trailhead by the silo and pick up the Ridge Trail. This all-access path of pea gravel makes a level track along the rim of the Colorado. Short spur trails lead to overlooks complete with contemplation benches. The Woodland Trail soon leaves left—this will be your return route. At just over 0.5 miles, the Valley View Trail leaves right, and ahead is yet another junction. Dead ahead is a vista point and the end of the Ridge Trail. Check out the

----

Directions

From the Austin airport take TX 71 east for 13.2 miles to reach McKinney Roughs Nature Park, on your left.

view and then drop onto the Bluff Trail Loop, which shortly splits. Stay right and keep downhill on a rocky trail with many switchbacks amid scattered cedars and oaks. Grasses and cacti thrive in places too.

At 1 mile, you'll bisect the Bluestem Trail. Ahead, the Bluff Trail Loop features four consecutive fenced overlooks, each better than the last. A shortcut to the Bluestem Trail is at the fourth overlook. Stay with the Bluff Trail Loop beyond the fourth overlook and come to the Bluestem Trail yet again. Now take the Bluestem Trail and drop off the hill you've been on to reach the Riverside Trail amid Colorado River bottomland, which is rife with hardwoods and lush grasses.

Turn left onto the Riverside Trail, working away from the river and around a wet-weather drainage. Reach Coyote Road at 1.5 miles. (You have only covered 1.5 miles after all those path intersections.) Coyote Road is open only to park personnel and is really a trail. Turn right here, and keep with Coyote Road as the Roadrunner Trail leaves left. Coyote Road is open overhead. Big cottonwoods grow along the Colorado River to your right. Not surprisingly, you'll reach another junction at nearly 2 miles. Turn right onto the Deep Sandy Trail. It comes nearer the river, rolling like a gentle roller coaster amid hackberry trees, sycamores, and tangled vines. Pass a little shortcut to Coyote Road. True to its name, the Deep Sandy trailbed is deep and sandy in spots. In other areas, the path bisects clearings.

At mile 2.5, a short spur leads down to a grass and gravel bar along the river. Walk directly to the water—upstream is an island. The Deep Sandy Trail then curves away from the river, passing a gated special events area to the right, then reaches Coyote Road again. Turn left here, beginning your return journey. Traverse a fence line amid large pecans before reaching the Pecan Bottom Trail at mile 3.3. Turn right here, enjoying the level, shady path as it heads toward a hillside. Look for narrow deer trails crisscrossing the bottomland. You won't miss the massive pecan tree—it would take at least two people with arms stretched to reach around it. Drift back toward the hillside once more before returning to Coyote Road at 4 miles. At this point, you will be backtracking a bit before covering new territory. Take Coyote Road, passing Roadrunner Trail and returning to Riverside Trail. Take the Riverside Trail and leave bottomland for good at the Bluestem Trail. Take the Bluestem Trail back to the Bluff Trail Loop. Turn right here and begin covering new terrain, working uphill and passing some stunning views. One grass meadow with a contemplation bench features sweeping views of Wilbargers Bend and beyond.

The Bluff Trail Loop ends to meet the Woodland Trail and the Ridge Trail. Take the Woodland Trail as it dips into thickets of trees and brush. A fantastic vista with a bench is reached just before intersecting the Ridge Trail at 5.5 miles. Turn right here and backtrack a short bit to the trailhead.

NEARBY ACTIVITIES

The Mark Rose Environmental Learning Center offers a variety of educational programs about the outdoors in general and McKinney Roughs in particular. They also have meeting facilities, a large dining room, and dorms.

ONION CREEK LOOP 07

IN BRIEF

Bikers, joggers, and hikers share this loop around McKinney Falls State Park as it winds through the shady banks of Onion Creek and past more ruins from Thomas McKinney's home.

DESCRIPTION

Explore enough of Austin's nearby trails and you will undoubtedly come across the name of Thomas F. McKinney. Like the Homestead Trail, Onion Creek Trail lies within McKinney Falls State Park, just inside the city limits.

In addition to establishing the area's first mill, McKinney also bred and raced horses on this land. The improvements here even included a private track, which wasn't the first one he ever built. While in Galveston, where he served in the state legislature, he also built a race course. After moving to the Austin area, he built another one here, across the river from the capital city.

Originally a league of land (about 5,700 acres), the remaining 744-acre state park contains numerous signs of the residence that once stood here. Although the gristmill and homestead ruins are found on the Homestead Trail, the remains of his horse trainer's cabin and long lines of stone fence remain on this path, and they even mark part of the park's boundary.

The hike begins at the Smith Visitor Center, where hikers can purchase bird checklists,

---

Directions ⟶

The park is located southeast of the state capitol in Austin off US 183. From US 183 take McKinney Falls Parkway 2.8 miles to the park.

ℹ KEY AT-A-GLANCE INFORMATION

LENGTH: 2.6 miles

CONFIGURATION: Loop

DIFFICULTY: Easy

SCENERY: Onion Creek, wildlife, wildflowers, and birds

EXPOSURE: Shady

TRAFFIC: Moderate

TRAIL SURFACE: Asphalt

HIKING TIME: Less than 1 hour

DRIVING DISTANCE: 10 miles from the state capitol

ACCESS: Daily, 8 a.m.–10 p.m. and overnight camping; $5 entrance fee/person over age 13

WHEELCHAIR ACCESS: Yes

MAPS: Available at park office or at tpwd.state.tx.us/publications

FACILITIES: Restrooms, showers, campsites, and park store

CONTACT INFORMATION: (512) 243-1643; tpwd.state.tx.us/spdest/findadest/parks/mckinney_falls

GPS TRAILHEAD COORDINATES

LATITUDE:: 30° 18' 32.78"
LONGITUDE: 97° 72' 56.39"

N

0   0.1   0.2
mile

McKINNEY FALLS
STATE PARK

Upper McKinney
Falls

Smith
Visitor Center

John Van
Hogen Cabin

park
headquarters

Onion Creek

McKinney Falls Pkwy.

diverge

Unofficial Upper Onion
Creek Trail

FEET

700
650
600
550
500
450
400
350
300

0.5   1   1.5   2   2.6

MILES

walking sticks, and other various items from the park staff. At a natural pool where the Big McKinney Falls area of Onion Creek is visible in front of the visitor center, swimmers create the only noise here. The trailhead is located on the south side of the building and is marked with a sign.

Watch for bicyclists as you walk down the path to the right, into the shady picnic area. The path is about 50 yards from the creek, and you'll see several picnic tables spread out under the tall trees. The first 0.4 miles snakes through the picnic and primitive camping areas of the park. At 0.5 miles, the woods get thick, and you get a little closer to the creek. Keep an eye out for the painted bunting, a small, colorful songbird that nests in the park through the summer. They are more abundant on the Homestead Trail but can still be seen here as well.

The trail passes by a stone embankment on the left that serves to prevent further erosion of the hillside. A small foot trail also leads down to the creek on the right. However, continue on the main path, which makes a steep climb as it turns to the left, away from the creek. A sign advises that bikers coming the other way walk their bikes at this point, but keep your eyes open anyway. At the top of the rise, a park bench offers a place to sit and rest or watch the birds.

About 1.2 miles into the hike, you'll see another bench off the trail as well as a stone wall that used to serve as the land's boundary. McKinney built the wall in the mid-1800s. A modern fence parallels the wall. The trail forks at 1.7 miles. Turn left and you will end up in the RV campsite area, so take the trail to the right. Not far from the fork you'll see an observation blind made of a wooden bench and wall. Across the trail in a clearing is a bird feeder. Avid birders can use this area, and the wall will allow them to set a spotting scope for close observation.

In the spring, large sections of the tall grass are pressed down by deer birthing their fawns. Attentive hikers can spy the fawns hiding under the bushes or hear them calling to their mothers. These babies are not lost and should be left alone. This is a common mistake made by people trying to help who actually wind up hurting the deer. Please take only pictures of the fawns.

More of the rock fence appears 2.2 miles along the path and still serves as the park boundary. Another bench located near here lets you sit and watch the passersby as well as the deer and birds. The park headquarters is visible through the trees to the right, as are the campsites to the left. The trail crosses the park road at 2.4 miles. Directly across the road are the ruins of the cabin that belonged to John Van Hogen, Thomas McKinney's horse trainer. Cross the road carefully to get a better look. You'll exit the woods after walking 2.6 miles and find yourself back at the Smith Visitor Center. The water fountain inside offers a cool drink, or you could immerse yourself in the creek.

NEARBY ACTIVITIES

The state park also offers camping, picnicking, mountain biking, swimming, and fishing.

08 PACE BEND TRAIL

KEY AT-A-GLANCE INFORMATION

LENGTH: 6 miles

CONFIGURATION: Out-and-back

DIFFICULTY: Moderate

SCENERY: Lake, woods, and grasslands

EXPOSURE: Moderate

TRAFFIC: Light

TRAIL SURFACE: Dirt

HIKING TIME: 3 hours

DRIVING DISTANCE: 33 miles from the state capitol

ACCESS: Daily, sunrise–sunset; $10 day-use fee/vehicle

MAPS: co.travis.tx.us/tnr/parks/pdf_files/pacebend.pdf

FACILITIES: None

CONTACT INFORMATION: (512) 264-1482; co.travis.tx.us/tnr/parks/pace_bend.asp

GPS TRAILHEAD COORDINATES

LATITUDE: : 30° 46' 61.11"
LONGITUDE: 98° 01' 50.83"

IN BRIEF

Although Pace Bend lacks interpretive information, its unattended and understated nature offers a great deal of appeal to hikers seeking peace and quiet. This place is definitely a well-kept secret for hiking.

DESCRIPTION

Located 30 miles west of Austin, the 1,368-acre Pace Bend Park is one of the more popular water recreation parks in the area. However, if you avoid the shorelines, regardless of the crowds, the solitude just might surprise you. The trails at Pace Bend are primarily little-used maintenance/jeep roads, providing a wide and easy-to-follow path for most of the hike. Wildlife or hikers who strayed from the established path have created numerous other trails, but the main trail is easy to discern from these.

The majority of the hike takes place between stands of trees. Plenty of open space overhead warrants a hat and sunscreen to prevent an otherwise great day from turning into a sunburned nightmare. It doesn't take long for the sun to work its magic, so take all necessary precautions. One other feature of the hike merits a mention: spiders. The arachnids around here are of the extra-large variety and are often found on large webs spanning the trails, so keep an eye out for them both in the air ahead and on the ground below (tarantulas are also prevalent).

- -

Directions ⟶

From the intersection of Texas Ranch Road 620 and TX 71, take TX 71 west 11 miles to RR 2322. Turn right on RR 2322 and travel 4.6 miles to the park entrance.

As you hike along the trail, keep your eyes on the tree lines when not watching for spiders, and you should see plenty of wildlife. The proximity of the trail to Lake Travis is a natural draw for mammals and waterfowl alike. Bring your birding binoculars, and you'll be treated to everything from titmice to pelicans, depending on the time of year. Songbirds and shorebirds populate this area.

The hike starts at the northernmost part of the park. Head south, and about a half mile from the trailhead you'll reach the first fork in the path. At this point, take the right fork. The hardest part of this hike is to know which forks to take to get the most out of what it has to offer. With that in mind, take a left at the next fork, and at the third fork, take a right. Just beyond this third fork is a T-intersection. The road to the left heads toward the lake and dead-ends into the main park road, so take the path to the right.

About 2 miles from the intersection, you'll come to a fenced-in area with a water tank and building on the inside. They appear to be in good shape and don't seem to have been abandoned. No other paths lead to it, however, so it remains a bit of a mystery. If you follow the fence around to the left, you'll find the trail. It leads southeast through a small creek valley and ends at a second trailhead on the main road that loops around the park. When you reach this point, turn back and return to the fenced area. When back at the fenced area, head left, and you should see another spur trail heading to the southwest. Take this path, which is a little rougher and overgrown than the rest of the trail. If you want to shorten the hike and you have two cars, a shuttle can be set at the end of this spur trail, which intersects the main loop road. Otherwise, return again to the fenced area.

At the fenced area, head left, where the foliage is sparser, offering good views of the water and the houses on the opposite bank. You will also notice several small trails leading to the left that you might want to investigate in the future, but for now, take your time and continue around the fenced area until you intersect the main trail. Turn left (north) and take your time looking for anything you might have missed on the way down.

PINE RIDGE LOOP 09

IN BRIEF

This hike explores the McKinney Roughs from high to low and back again. Start along a high plateau to circle around and down to the Colorado River, gaining far-reaching views from the plateau rim. Cruise beside the wide-water course to return via a trail that offers more views. Old homesites and ranch relics can be seen along the way.

DESCRIPTION

In 1995 the Lower Colorado River Authority (LCRA) acquired the land now known as McKinney Roughs and built a first-rate environmental education facility to complement a 1,100-acre preserve along the Colorado River between Austin and Bastrop. Today, the park has 18 miles of hiking and equestrian trails that explore the rugged terrain, which earned the name *roughs* from the vertical variation that made large-scale agriculture difficult. The steep ravines and thick woods also provided refuge for frontier outlaws.

The park trailhead is a short walk toward the metal silo beside the park office. Find the marked Riverside Trail and follow a partly wooded plateau environment dominated by cedar trees. At 0.2 miles you'll reach a trail intersection. Keep forward, now on Pine Ridge Trail. (Fox Tail Trail leaves to the right, and Riverside Trail continues left. Riverside Trail to your left will be your return route.)

Pine Ridge Trail cruises along the rim of the Colorado River Valley, passing Bobcat

----

Directions —————————————→

From the Austin airport take TX 71 east for 13.2 miles to reach McKinney Roughs Nature Park, on the left.

KEY AT-A-GLANCE INFORMATION

LENGTH: 4.1 miles

CONFIGURATION: Loop

DIFFICULTY: Moderate

SCENERY: River bluffs, pine–oak woodlands

EXPOSURE: Half shady, half sunny

TRAFFIC: Moderate

TRAIL SURFACE: Dirt, leaves, pine needles

HIKING TIME: 2.25 hours

DRIVING DISTANCE: 24 miles from the state capitol

ACCESS: Monday–Saturday, 8 a.m.–5 p.m.; Sunday, noon–5 p.m.; $4 entrance fee/person over age 13

WHEELCHAIR ACCESS: Yes, at hike's beginning

MAPS: lcra.org/library/media/ public/docs/community/ community_mck_roughs_trailmap .pdf

FACILITIES: Picnic area, restroom at park office

CONTACT INFORMATION: (512) 303-5073; lcra.org/parks/developed_ parks/mckinney_roughs.html

GPS TRAILHEAD COORDINATES

LATITUDE: : 30° 14' 26.94"
LONGITUDE: 97° 45' 72.22"

Ridge Trail at just over 0.5 miles. Scattered woodlands break up clearings where cacti sporadically reach above the grass. Ahead, Pond Spur Trail leaves right to an old stock pond. Large loblolly pines grow in the area. Pass through more clearings, keeping your eyes peeled for remains of an old homestead chimney. A crumbling barn is more evident directly beside the trail.

McKinney Roughs has been home to humans for a long time. Aboriginal Texans lived in the area as long as 8,000 years ago. They ate what the land allowed, cooking acorns and cacti in limestone-slab ovens. Oven remnants helped archaeologists place them here. Later, bows and arrows enabled meat to become more common fare. Their way of life went downhill when European explorers came this way in the 1500s. Then, in the early 1820s, Stephen F. Austin and his band of settlers arrived. One of them was Thomas F. McKinney, for whom the area was named, though he lived 12 miles distant. A fellow named John Calhoun Wise settled here in the 1850s. His descendants stayed another 100 years. Ultimately the land was obtained by the LCRA, and you and I can enjoy it today.

Pine Ridge Trail continues along the rim and then traverses a knife-edge ridgeline widening to a little knob. Circle around the knob to reach a contemplation bench and a far-reaching view of the Colorado River Valley at just over 2 miles. Take in the vista before beginning your descent toward the Colorado River by switchbacks on cedar steps. Reach a streambed and follow it a bit, crossing the branch on a bridge, and ascend to intersect the Cypress Trail at 2.5 miles. Note the clay erosion-created ravines on the way up.

Now take Cypress Trail down beneath thick woods to reach the riparian zone along the Colorado. Walk among the moisture-loving hardwoods—sycamore, cottonwood, and hackberry. Hackberry trees are identified by their warty gray bark.

Cypress Trail travels upstream along the Colorado. Exit Cypress Trail and join Riverside Trail at just over 3 miles. Turn left here on the wide path open to hikers and equestrians. As you climb the hill away from the river, turn around to enjoy more views of the lands beyond the Colorado. The land on the far side of the river encompasses Wilbargers Bend. Pass the Bluestem Trail coming in from your right.

Bobcat Ridge Trail comes in from your left on reaching the plateau above the river. Enjoy the level stroll after your climb. The path is open to the sun overhead as it makes its way through grass clearings and scattered brush and cedar coppices topped with ever-present oaks. Valley View Trail comes in from your right at 3.6 miles. Keep cruising along the plateau to reach a final trail junction. Riverside Trail turns right here. Retrace your steps 0.2 miles to return to the trailhead.

NEARBY ACTIVITIES

The Mark Rose Environmental Learning Center offers a variety of educational programs about the outdoors in general and McKinney Roughs in particular. They also have meeting facilities, a large dining room, and dorms.

10   SCULPTURE FALLS HIKE AT BARTON CREEK

KEY AT-A-GLANCE INFORMATION

LENGTH: 3 miles

CONFIGURATION: Out-and-back

DIFFICULTY: Moderate

SCENERY: River canyon, waterfalls, rich woods

EXPOSURE: Mostly shady

TRAFFIC: Very heavy

TRAIL SURFACE: Dirt, rock

HIKING TIME: 2.5 hours

DRIVING DISTANCE: 7 miles from the state capitol

ACCESS: Daily, 5 a.m.–10 p.m.; no fees or permits

WHEELCHAIR ACCESS: No

MAPS: ci.austin.tx.us/parks/ parkdirectory.htm

FACILITIES: None

CONTACT INFORMATION: (512) 974-6700; ci.austin.tx.us/parks

GPS TRAILHEAD COORDINATES

LATITUDE:: 30° 24' 40.56"
LONGITUDE: 97° 81' 04.72"

IN BRIEF

This out-and-back hike begins midway along the Barton Creek Greenbelt. Leave the busy Twin Falls–Gaines Access and descend into the Barton Creek canyon. Once in the canyon, head upstream, passing Twin Falls before reaching Sculpture Falls. The deep pools by both falls make for alluring swimming holes.

DESCRIPTION

The Barton Creek Greenbelt is one of Austin's outdoor treasures and is enjoyed by an abundance of outdoor enthusiasts, not only to hike but also to rock climb, mountain bike, and swim. This particular section of the Greenbelt has two waterfalls and swimming holes, making it very popular. It may be the busiest stretch of trail in this entire guidebook. So when you come here, try to make it during the week. In the morning would be even better. The often-busy trail leaves the often-busy MoPac Highway, cruising along the rim of the canyon before angling down toward Barton Creek. The first waterfall, Twin Falls, is shortly upstream. Keep forward, traveling beneath tunnel-like woods to reach Sculpture Falls, another wide drop over a rock shelf.

The trailhead has a signboard to help orient you. Pass the signboard and walk a few

---

Directions

From MoPac, Loop 1, south of the Colorado River, take the exit for Loop 360 south, Capital of Texas Highway. After getting off MoPac, keep south on the frontage road rather than actually getting on Loop 360 north or south. The Twin Falls–Gaines Access is on the right side of the frontage road before it loops back under MoPac.

Scottish Woods Trail

Sculpture Falls

360

Walsh Tarlton Lane

Capital of TX Hwy.

Barton Creek

frontage road

MoPac Expressway

BARTON CREEK WILDERNESS PARK

Twin Falls

Twin Falls–
Gaines Access

360

frontage road

Barton Creek

MoPac Expressway

700
650
600
550
500
450
400
350
300

FEET

0.25   0.5   0.75   1   1.25   1.5

MILES

steps to the rim of the canyon. Cedar trees collectively shade the dirt path. Head right, upstream, though Barton Creek is far below. Shortly descend on a graded trail to reach a post at 0.2 miles. The trees are much thicker and taller here in the riverine woodland of the canyon.

Clear-blue Barton Creek flows on your left. Head upstream. You will notice how the heavily used path braids into numerous paths cut by multiple users. Twin Falls is just ahead. Here, the creek gets backed up before collecting energy and then pushing over a rock shelf in two different channels to make deep pools. The pool closest to the trail is very popular with swimmers escaping the heat of a Texas summer.

Keep upstream, passing a gray and tan bluff. Look for eroded overhangs and grottoes in the bluff walls. Small riffles and shoals noisily accompany hikers. Live oaks and cedars grow seemingly everywhere but the trail, forming a tunnel around the path. Pass a normally dry feeder branch coming in from your right. Past this point, look for a stone fence coursing through the woods. This fence runs roughly parallel to the creek and is part of a group of walls, circles, and other formations. Local legend has it that these rock formations were part of a failed Spanish mission from the early 1700s.

Here, the trail really splits apart. Side trails lead down to the creek; others lead into the woods away from the water. Others run side by side up the canyon. Pick your route, whether it goes through the deep woods or along the stream.

Reach Sculpture Falls at 1.5 miles. Barton Creek descends over a dimpled shelf of rock. A long, deep pool forms below the low, wide drop. The rock shelf continues on the far side of the stream. If you can rock-hop over there, the shelf makes for an excellent relaxing spot for lunch or sunbathing—or simply to toss your shoes off and take a dip.

From Sculpture Falls, the Barton Creek Greenbelt continues 1.3 miles farther, ending with a climb up a steep hill known as the Trail of Life. The hill climbs 300 feet in 0.3 miles, ending at a neighborhood off Scottish Woods Trail. This trailhead is known as the Camp Craft Access. The many No Parking signs around the trailhead make leaving a car here a risky endeavor. Your best bet is to make this an out-and-back hike, whether you go to trail's end or not.

NEARBY ACTIVITIES

This section of the Barton Creek Greenbelt offers mountain biking, swimming, and rock climbing.

SHOAL CREEK GREENBELT

IN BRIEF

This trek along a downtown Austin Greenbelt path heads up the watershed of Shoal Creek, passing through several urban parks before ending just beyond an overhanging bluff, 25 city blocks away. The mix of city scenery, stone trail work, and the nature of Shoal Creek combine to provide a getaway not only for hikers but also for bikers and runners.

DESCRIPTION

An urban greenbelt can only get so woodsy. Austin's city planners did a good job with the Shoal Creek Greenbelt, creating a pathway that used already-existing parks and connecting them using the narrow strip of land along Shoal Creek. Start this trek at Duncan Park off Ninth Street, and then head up to 31st Street, nearing House Park and passing through Pease Park and Dog Park. Short portions of the trail exist on both ends beyond this stretch, but each end currently has problems. The trail between Duncan Park and Town Lake is still not connected, and the part north of 31st Street travels along a street for a distance before petering out altogether. Both ends may be extended and completed in the future, but for now the following section is the best the trail offers.

KEY AT-A-GLANCE INFORMATION

LENGTH: 5 miles

CONFIGURATION: Out-and-back

DIFFICULTY: Moderate

SCENERY: Wooded city parks, urban creek, scattered forest

EXPOSURE: Partly sunny, partly shady

TRAFFIC: Moderate to heavy

TRAIL SURFACE: Rock, pea gravel, dirt

HIKING TIME: 2.75 hours

DRIVING DISTANCE: 1 mile from state capitol

ACCESS: Daily, 5 a.m.–10 p.m.; no fees or permits

WHEELCHAIR ACCESS: Yes

MAPS: ci.austin.tx.us/parks/parkdirectory.htm

FACILITIES: Water fountain, restroom at Pease Park

CONTACT INFORMATION: (512) 974-6700; ci.austin.tx.us/parks

Directions

From I-35 take Exit 234B, Eighth–Third Streets, and then take the frontage road to Sixth Street. Head west on Sixth Street for 1 mile to West Avenue. Turn right on West Avenue and follow it three blocks to Ninth Street. Turn left on Ninth Street. Duncan Park is on your right. Park on the street by the park. Take the Shoal Creek Greenbelt north, heading upstream along the creek from Duncan Park.

GPS TRAILHEAD COORDINATES

LATITUDE: : 30° 27' 35.28"
LONGITUDE: 97° 75' 13.61"

29th St.

31st St.

creek crossing
(no bridge)

29th St.

(Note: Dog park is between
24th St. and 29th St.)

**DOG
PARK**

Windsor Rd.

Lamar Blvd.

24th St.

Shoal Creek

MLK Blvd.

**PEASE
PARK**

15th St.

**HOUSE
PARK**

Austin
Recreation Center

12th St.

Windsor Rd.

9th St.

**DUNCAN
PARK**

N

0   0.1   0.2
mile

FEET

700
650
600
550
500
450
400
350
300

0.5   1   1.5   2   2.5

MILES

City dwellers can be seen running, biking, or walking dogs along this trail. It is also used as a handy north–south connector for downtown pedestrians. From Ninth Street, begin heading north on the pebbled concrete path east of Shoal Creek. A live oak tree shades the trail entrance. A sign gives the address, 900 West Ninth Street. Across the road to the south is a bike track. Duncan Park is a rolling, grassy expanse dotted with trees and benches. Pass under the 10th Street Bridge, the first of many bridge underpasses, and keep along a green corridor bordered with stonework to stabilize the trail.

Ahead, across Shoal Creek Boulevard, are House Park and the Austin Recreation Center. Willow, live oak, and brush line Shoal Creek. At just over 0.5 miles, span Shoal Creek on an iron trestle bridge to enter Pease Park. The trail is pea gravel now and divides into two sections here, each circling around the lower end of Pease Park, established in 1875 on land bought by the sitting Texas Governor Elisha Pease. A small swimming pool and large playground occupy much of the lower end of the park. A water fountain is beside the pool, and a restroom is on the far side of the play area, on the left-hand trail passing through the park.

The primary path keeps forward through Pease Park to rejoin the left trail just before ascending a cedar-covered hill. Dip from the hill and come alongside Shoal Creek again in a floodplain. By now you have noticed the metal-and-chain holes for a disc golf course in the park. Also look for a streamside live oak tree that leans down current. During its long life, periodic floods have sculpted the tree to grow that way.

The Shoal Creek Greenbelt now passes under 24th Street. Enter Dog Park, where pet owners are allowed to let their dogs roam without a leash. Watch your feet here, as well as in the surrounding wooded floodplain. The trail shortly crosses Shoal Creek Boulevard, at this point not much more than a quiet park road. A hill to your left and the creek to your right pinch the pathway, until the trail is forced to cross Shoal Creek at just over 2 miles. There is no bridge. Shortly pass under 29th Street, coming to the most scenic part of the path. A craggy, dark bluff rises to the right of the way. Boulders have fallen off the bluff, creating a mosaic of rocks dotted with ferns and moss. The trail abuts the bluff and then travels under the overhang on a section that is sheer enough to require handrails. Suddenly turn away from the creek and emerge onto 31st Street, a vastly different scene than what you've just passed through. This is a good turnaround point.

If you want to continue on the trail, turn left and follow 31st Street past houses, then dive left into the creek bed on a pebbled concrete path. The trail continues along Shoal Creek to just beyond 38th Street for the time being; with any luck, it will be finished in the future.

NEARBY ACTIVITIES

Pease Park is the most developed park along the Shoal Creek Greenbelt, with play areas, picnic tables, and a disc golf course.

12 SLAUGHTER CREEK TRAIL

KEY AT-A-GLANCE INFORMATION

LENGTH: 2.4 miles

CONFIGURATION: Loop

DIFFICULTY: Easy

SCENERY: Public park play-scapes, Slaughter Creek, birds and wildlife, and a karst

EXPOSURE: Moderate

TRAFFIC: Moderate

TRAIL SURFACE: Gravel, dirt, concrete

HIKING TIME: 1.5 hours

DRIVING DISTANCE: 11 miles from the state capitol

ACCESS: Daily, 24 hours; no entrance fee

WHEELCHAIR ACCESS: No

MAPS: None

FACILITIES: None

CONTACT INFORMATION: (512) 974-6700; ci.austin.tx.us/parks

GPS TRAILHEAD COORDINATES

LATITUDE:: 30° 20' 17.50"
LONGITUDE: 97° 88' 43.06"

IN BRIEF

Although located in a milder park environment, this trail offers some rougher terrain as well as a very interesting geological feature. If you don't know what karst is, this hike will fill in the gaps for you.

DESCRIPTION

The trails in the 546-acre Slaughter Creek Park are mainly large loops around the soccer fields. The paved Veloway is only for bikes and in-line skates. The other trails are primarily used for jogging and walking by local residents; it is useful for a change of scenery, or even change of pace, from some of the more strenuous trails in the area. Much of the hike takes place on a wide jeep trail, and this is where the walk starts. In the beginning the trail leads both left and right. Go left down the jeep trail to begin, and you'll return from the right when you've completed the loop.

The trail continues in an almost straight path for about 0.75 miles, at which point you'll make a turn to the right with the path. When you reach the creek, you'll see another jeep road crossing it, but the one you're on doesn't appear to continue on the other side. Another trail here heads toward the creek, and this is the trail you will take. When you reach the creek, you'll cross it. A concrete walkway crosses the creek, so getting over the water is no problem at all. Here and at most points of the hike, you are within sight and earshot of the soccer fields. On game days,

----

Directions ⟶

Head south on MoPac, take the Slaughter Lane exit, and head west. The parking area is on the left side of the road, and the park is on the right.

N

0   0.1   0.2

mile

To MoPac Expressway

W. Slaughter Lane

Escarpment Boulevard

Slaughter Creek

soccer field

soccer field

soccer field

soccer field

soccer field

soccer field

soccer field

rough, rocky terrain

La Crosse Avenue

maintenance road

FEET

1,000
950
900
850
800
750
700
650
600

0.5   1   1.5   2   2.4

MILES

the solace of the park will not be as evident as it is during off-peak hours. Because many teams and leagues use the facilities, there is no real way to know ahead of time when it will be in use.

The trail continues west now for about 0.5 miles along the crushed-gravel perimeter of the soccer complex and then turns north back toward the trailhead. Shortly after this turn, you'll see a chain-link fence near one of the soccer fields and a play-scape. If you investigate a little closer, you'll see a hole in the ground on the other side. This, however, is not just a hole—it is a karst.

A karst is a sink, or cave, formed by underground streams that dissolve the rock beneath the surface. The water supply in karsts is very susceptible to contamination. This is one reason for the fence. The other reason is more obvious: to protect people from falling into the hole. Whatever your reason, don't cross the fence.

When you've finished examining this geological feature, continue back toward the trailhead. When you do reach it, turn left, taking the trail you passed at the beginning of the hike. The jeep road disappears about 0.2 miles past the trailhead and becomes extremely rocky—be careful so you won't be too rough on your ankles. When you reach the next creek crossing, you won't find another concrete walkway. You'll have to negotiate it by hopping across on the rocks (and there's something about doing this that just brings out the kid in everyone).

From here, the trail hugs the sideline of a soccer field but then continues straight back along a fence and maintenance trail. This area is currently being built up and will change a great deal in the years to come. When you reach a point where you really can go no farther, turn back, play at the creek crossing again, even skip a stone or two, and make your way back to the trailhead. If a game is on, and you like soccer, stick around.

Though by no means difficult, this hike is ideal for beginners or for a weekday evening when you just have to get outside and don't feel like doing yard work.

SPICEWOOD VALLEY TRAIL 13

IN BRIEF

This suburban jewel of a hike is tucked away in a deeply wooded canyon, where a tributary of Bull Creek flows through a bluff-bordered forest corridor. The shady trek enters the canyon, passing by spring branches, under big trees, and astride an old homesite. Toward the end, spur paths connect to neighboring Mountain View Park and the adjacent Scotland Wells neighborhood.

DESCRIPTION

This green trail corridor, set in suburban hills north of downtown Austin, is so hidden from view that I bet many nearby residents don't even know it's there. The Spicewood Valley Trail, developed in late 2005, isn't very well marked or publicized but serves as an example of how to integrate quality wilderness-type paths into a populated area.

The hike traces a tributary of Bull Creek as the feeder branch cuts a startlingly steep canyon. Cedars shade the path for much of the way. In other areas, especially the flats along the creek, live oaks provide protection from sun. Just as with other areas distant from downtown Austin, this was once ranch country. You will find relics of a small operation, from the home foundation to a spring to a small tributary dam. Nearby, a remnant field hangs on as trees continually reclaim the flat. Farther

----

Directions ━━━━━━━━━━━━━━━━━━━━━━━━━━▶

From US 183 north of Loop 360 north of downtown Austin, take the Spicewood Springs Road westerly (McNeil Road leaves easterly here) for 1.8 miles to Scotland Well Drive, at the bottom of a hill. Turn right on Scotland Well Drive, and the parking area is immediately on your right.

KEY AT-A-GLANCE INFORMATION

LENGTH: 2.6 miles

CONFIGURATION: Out-and-back

DIFFICULTY: Easy

SCENERY: Wooded creek valley

EXPOSURE: Shady

TRAFFIC: Moderate

TRAIL SURFACE: Natural surfaces

HIKING TIME: 1.5 hours

DRIVING DISTANCE: 16 miles from the state capitol

ACCESS: Daily, 5 a.m.–10 p.m.; no fees or permits

WHEELCHAIR ACCESS: None

MAPS: ci.austin.tx.us/parks/parkdirectory.htm

FACILITIES: Mountain View Park has a short path, restrooms, and picnic areas.

CONTACT INFORMATION: (512) 974-6700; ci.austin.tx.us/parks

GPS TRAILHEAD COORDINATES

LATITUDE: : 30° 25' 22.05"
LONGITUDE: 97° 47' 38.05"

N

| 0 | 0.1 | 0.2 |

mile

Balcones
Country Club
Lake

cascade

Evening Primrose Path

Topridge Drive

Middlebie
Drive

Westerkirk Drive

Scotland Well Drive

MOUNTAIN
VIEW
PARK

P

Callanish Park Drive

Tweed Berwick Drive

Ashton Ridge

Marybank Drive

Scotsman Drive

old homesite

Scotland Well Drive

Spicewood Springs Road

P

Bintliff Drive

Old Lampasas Trail

FEET

900						
850						
800						
750						
700						
650						
600						
550						
500						

| 0.25 | 0.5 | 0.75 | 1 | 1.3 |

MILES

Overhanging bluffs border the trail.

upstream, the trail bisects springs that feed the main tributary. Later the canyon closes in and rock bluffs squeeze the path, which finally ends just downstream from a watery cascade. On this upper end of the trail, there are two alternate trailheads, which is a good thing because the main trailhead on Scotland Well Drive has limited parking. If the Scotland Well lot is full, continue on Scotland Well Drive for 0.6 miles to Westerkirk Drive. Turn right on Westerkirk Drive and follow it to a parking area on the left at Mountain View Park. From here, you pick up the trail by walking east through the small park to Callanish Park Drive. Look for the trail descending easterly between two houses on Callanish Park Drive.

From the Scotland Well trailhead, begin your trek by joining the sidewalk uphill 300 feet along Scotland Well Drive and then bearing right into a tunnel of cedar on a marked gravel track about 4 feet wide. Step over a few intermittent drainages on the well-shaded steep slope. Stone and cedar supports keep the trail level and non-erosive. At 0.3 miles a user-created path cuts right, south, back to the parking lot along the tributary. The trail opens to an alluring meadow with the remains of a jalopy down by the creek. The valley closes and trees reign again, including sycamores. At 0.6 miles pass a concrete box spring on your left. Just ahead, look left for the foundation of a house. The homesite was well placed. It is near ample level land and is on the west side of the canyon, protecting it from the afternoon heat of the long central Texas summer. Note the ornamental vegetation beside the homesite, where a pair of chimneys are outlined. Just ahead a dam spans the small but clear stream. A resting bench lures hikers to relax and listen to the water spill.

At 0.9 miles the trail reaches a transitional meadow. Eventually the grassy area will be completely covered in trees. The Spicewood Valley Trail continues upstream, traveling the margin between the stream and meadow. At 1 mile you'll reach a trail junction. Here a spur trail leads left, angling up past piled stones and slicing through rocky bluffs to Callanish Drive and Mountain View Park. The main path keeps straight, crossing a couple of spring branches flowing from rugged terrain on the trail's left. The bluffs close in—you can see houses atop them through the trees. I wonder what the early homesteader would think of the suburban neighborhoods atop the canyon. Climb away from the flats angling up the left side of the bluffs. Travel alongside rock overhangs. Make a fat man's squeeze between the bluff and a fallen rock. Reach another trail junction at 1.2 miles. Here stone steps leave left uphill and emerge at the intersection of Topridge Drive and Evening Primrose Path. A user-created trail keeps forward and then shortly fades out above a cascade falling from a rock bluff. Unfortunately, this is the trail end and where you must backtrack.

NEARBY ACTIVITIES

Mountain View Park has shaded picnic facilities, a short hard-surface trail, and playgrounds.

TOWN LAKE TRAIL 14

IN BRIEF

This is by far the best-known and, as a direct result, the busiest trail in the Austin area. Hikers, bikers, and meanderers alike share this trail located in the heart of the state's capital. Watch kayakers and boaters play in the water while viewing some of the official buildings of the political center of Texas.

DESCRIPTION

To begin the loop around the lake, hike east, though you will have opportunities to turn around if the hike proves to be too long. As you walk, you're heading toward the heart of Zilker Park. Along the way you'll be able to see the park's soccer fields to your right, and you'll cross the narrow-gauge railroad tracks used by the popular Zilker Train.

The tree cover increases at this point and stays with you for a while, as you make your way to the confluence of Barton Springs and Town Lake. When you reach this point, you'll find a gazebo and a water fountain if you feel like taking a rest. There is also a good stretch of shoreline for interacting with some of the not-so-wild life. If you have some older bread lying around the house, bring it along to share with the ducks here. They'll appreciate it, and it's good for taking your mind off other things as well.

When you're finished at the gazebo, the trail turns south, along Barton Springs, and makes its way to an arched footbridge that

----

Directions ———————————————▶

The hike begins under the MoPac bridge, which is obviously located right off MoPac. Other parking is available, but this is the most convenient.

KEY AT-A-GLANCE INFORMATION

LENGTH: 7.2 miles

CONFIGURATION: Loop

DIFFICULTY: Easy

SCENERY: Lake, capitol building, and abundant greenery

EXPOSURE: Open–shady

TRAFFIC: Heavy

TRAIL SURFACE: Paved

HIKING TIME: 3 hours

DRIVING DISTANCE: One mile from the state capitol

ACCESS: Daily, 5 a.m.–10 p.m.; no fees or permits

WHEELCHAIR ACCESS: Yes

MAPS: None

FACILITIES: Restrooms

CONTACT INFORMATION: (512) 974-6700; ci.austin.tx.us/parks

GPS TRAILHEAD COORDINATES

LATITUDE: : 30° 27' 49.44"
LONGITUDE: 97° 77' 14.72"

crosses the tributary before heading back north to the lake. When you reach the lake again, the path turns right and makes its way toward Lamar Boulevard. The bridge crossing the road makes it easier for hikers to get across.

The park area at this point is known as Auditorium Shores and is the location of several concerts and events each year. Austinites love their music, and this is only one of many outdoor venues available to enjoy it. Along this section of the trail stands a statue of one of Austin's favorite sons. Stevie Ray Vaughn's guitar style took the music world by storm, and his brilliant career was cut tragically short in a helicopter accident.

You've hiked roughly 2 miles at this point, and it is a good place to turn back if you want to cut things short. If not, keep heading east toward Congress Avenue. Once you've crossed it, the trail runs into an apartment complex, but the hike doesn't have to end. Keep making your way toward Riverside Drive and I-35. The sidewalk here is right next to the road, and the motorists are less aware of you than you are of them. Use caution because they aren't driving particularly slowly. This is also where you'll encounter the steepest incline in the hike. Persevere through this less-than-peaceful area because the payoff is worth it.

Right before you reach I-35, a dog park can be seen on the left, where people can let their canine companions roam free of their leashes. This is another good spot for a break if Fido has been tugging on your arm for the past 3 miles. While resting, look ahead toward the interstate and you'll notice the separate pedestrian bridge that crosses Town Lake. When you're ready, this is how you'll get to the other side.

Once across the lake, the setting turns back to a more natural environment of trees and grass, and the traffic here is some of the lightest that you'll encounter. About 0.5 miles from the crossing, you'll reach a couple of interesting historical markers along the trail. The first marks the spot of the headquarters of the fifth military district after the Civil War. The second one, if taken at face value, is where barbed wire was first put to use.

Once you've crossed under Congress Avenue again, the foot and bike traffic increases but remains much more pleasant than the vehicular traffic of I-35. You may explore numerous side trails along the lake. One of them, Shoal Creek, is included in this book.

As you're nearing MoPac again, you'll see a large concrete and iron tower. This was part of a facility used to ferry clay over from the south side of the Colorado River, long before this became a recreational area.

Once you reach MoPac, cross over the lake on the pedestrian bridge and make your way to your car, or take on the Shoal Creek hike before calling it a day, if you have the energy and the inclination to do so.

15 TURKEY CREEK TRAIL

IN BRIEF

Emma Long Metropolitan Park is the setting for this hike. Travel up the canyon of Turkey Creek, where the path crosses the clear waters of Turkey Creek numerous times. The fern wall of the creek canyon is a highlight before the trail leaves the canyon, traversing the rim on its return journey.

DESCRIPTION

This fun trail explores the lush canyon of Turkey Creek, where cedars, oaks, and sycamores form a nearly continuous tree canopy. Sheer rock bluffs and sloping, wooded walls lead down to crystal-clear Turkey Creek. Leave the parking area and immediately enter a grove of cedar trees with their interconnected branches forming a dark canopy. The forest floor is littered with rocks mixed with grass and brush. Drop to cross Turkey Creek near City Park Road. This is the first of numerous creek crossings, which can be easily made in times of normal flow. However, if you can't make the first rock-hop, turn back. Seventeen more such crossings await.

Turn upstream, passing an attractive picnic area. The sky penetrates the canyon in places, lighting occasional stream pools. The deeper pools have a bluish cast. Take a close look and see how easily you can peer into the clear water. In other places, Turkey Creek

---

KEY AT-A-GLANCE INFORMATION

LENGTH: 2.5 miles

CONFIGURATION: Balloon

DIFFICULTY: Moderate

SCENERY: Wooded creek canyon

EXPOSURE: Mostly shady

TRAFFIC: Moderate, busy on warm weekends

TRAIL SURFACE: Cedar shavings, rocks, dirt

HIKING TIME: 1.25 hours

DRIVING DISTANCE: 16 miles from the state capitol

ACCESS: Daily, 7 a.m.–10 p.m.; Monday–Thursday, $5 entrance fee/vehicle; Friday–Sunday and holidays, $8 entrance fee/vehicle

WHEELCHAIR ACCESS: No

MAPS: Available at park fee station 1 mile beyond trailhead or at ci.austin.tx.us/parks/parkdirectory.htm

FACILITIES: Water, restrooms at main park area on Lake Austin, picnic area near trailhead

CONTACT INFORMATION: (512) 974-6700; ci.austin.tx.us/parks

GPS TRAILHEAD COORDINATES

LATITUDE: : 30° 33' 21.67"
LONGITUDE: 97° 83' 74.44"

Directions

From MoPac, Loop Road 1, take FM 2222/Northland Drive west for 4.1 miles to City Park Road. Turn left on City Park Road, and travel 4.8 miles to the trailhead. The trailhead is 0.3 miles past a yellow park gate and then just past the bridge over Turkey Creek, on the right.

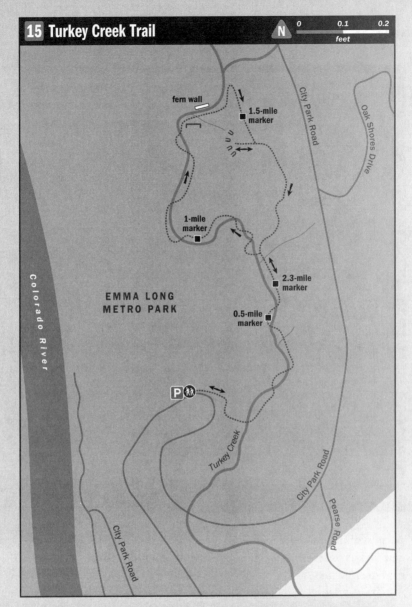

N

0   0.1   0.2
feet

fern wall

1.5-mile
marker

City Park Road

Oak Shores Drive

1-mile
marker

2.3-mile
marker

EMMA LONG
METRO PARK

0.5-mile
marker

Colorado River

P

Turkey Creek

City Park Road

City Park Road

Pearse Road

900
850
800
750
700
650
600
550
500

FEET

0.5   1   1.5   2   2.5
MILES

Turkey Creek

glides shallow and swift over wide rock flats. Small cascades offer an inviting visual and audio appeal to the walk. The narrowness of the canyon lends an intimate wilderness feel. The canyon walls alternately lower where dry washes feed into the main creek canyon.

The fords come frequently. On most crossings, natural stepping-stones have been laid across the creek. After the fourth crossing, you will reach the half-mile marker—it's literally a marker that tells you how far you've walked. Cross one more time before reaching the loop portion of the Turkey Creek Trail. Leave left, immediately crossing Turkey Creek, and then cross three more times before reaching the 1-mile marker on the inside of a stream curve.

The canyon widens, and the forest opens somewhat. Above, rocks and boulders are sprinkled on the hillsides. In other places, the canyon wall is plainly visible. Three more creek crossings lead you to the fern wall. Here, the moist and cool canyon wall supports a fern colony, resulting in a draping green swath hanging over the creek bed. A contemplation bench enhances the setting, allowing you to absorb the atmosphere of this lush locale. Look for moss growing on the horizontal branches of live oaks as more evidence of this green abundance.

Beyond the fern wall, turn away from Turkey Creek to ascend the side of the canyon. Here, the forest immediately has a more arid look. Scattered cedars grow their limbs down to ground level, side by side with grasses and limestone. Take a closer look at the rock and see how it has eroded into sharp edges in many spots. The sharp rock made me glad that I wasn't wearing sandals. Cacti take their place in the level areas of the canyon rim as well.

Pass the 1.5-mile marker and then reach a side trail leaving to the right. Take this short path to the edge of the canyon. Here, you can look down on the forest below, noting the wooded swale indicating the canyon depth and location. The trail walking is easy now and drifts closer to the canyon rim, ultimately descending a rocky path back down to Turkey Creek. The downhill trail is broken by cut cedar logs that prevent erosion and add steps, making the walk easier.

End the loop portion of the Turkey Creek Trail, backtracking downstream, making the stream crossings again. Pass the 2-mile marker and then the 2.5-mile marker. Make the final of the 18 creek crossings, returning to the trailhead.

NEARBY ACTIVITIES

This city park offers picnicking, camping, fishing, boating, and swimming.

16 WALLER CREEK GREENBELT

KEY AT-A-GLANCE INFORMATION

LENGTH: 2 miles

CONFIGURATION: Out-and-back

DIFFICULTY: Easy

SCENERY: Creek, stone bridges, urban buildings

EXPOSURE: Mostly open

TRAFFIC: Moderate–heavy

TRAIL SURFACE: Stones, concrete, pea gravel

HIKING TIME: 1.2 hours

DRIVING DISTANCE: Adjacent to state capitol

ACCESS: Daily, 5 a.m.–10 p.m.; no fees or permits

WHEELCHAIR ACCESS: Yes, except where stone steps occur

MAPS: ci.austin.tx.us/parks/ parkdirectory.htm

FACILITIES: None

CONTACT INFORMATION: (512) 974-6700; ci.austin.tx.us/parks

GPS TRAILHEAD COORDINATES

LATITUDE:: 30° 27' 60.28"
LONGITUDE: 97° 73' 55.00"

IN BRIEF

This urban greenbelt travels through downtown Austin. The stone walkway bridges Waller Creek numerous times on its southbound journey from Waterloo Park near the University of Texas (UT) campus down to Fifth Street. Even though this is an out-and-back hike, multiple parallel paths along Waller Creek can add variety to the walk.

DESCRIPTION

This is not a dirt path through the woods. It is instead an amazing amount of stonework in and around the bed of Waller Creek, which flows through downtown Austin. The city has done a lot to make this trail work, as it snakes below and between many buildings, streets, and businesses. Plans are afoot to turn this trail into a bona fide river walk, à la San Antonio. Take your time, and appreciate the numerous bridges and trail underpasses. Waller Creek is never far away, so, if the rains have been pouring, stay off this flood-prone path.

Pick up the Waller Creek Greenbelt near the corner of 15th Street and Red River Road. The trailhead is at the north end of Waterloo Park near the Ronald McDonald House. This city park has a little green space and picnic tables in addition to the Waller Creek Greenbelt. Stone steps flanked by stone walls descend

---

Directions

From I-35 take Exit 235, University of Texas/ MLK and 15th Street. Head east on 15th Street and follow it 0.2 miles toward the university campus to reach Red River Road. Turn left on Red River Road and park on the street next to Waterloo Park. On weekends you can park in any of the nearby state parking lots for free.

N

0   0.1   0.2
mile

15th St.

Waller Creek

STATE CAPITOL
COMPLEX

12th St.

WATERLOO
PARK

Red River Rd.

frontage road

35

11th St.

10th St.

9th St.

8th St.

7th St.

Trinity St.

Neches St.

Red River Rd.

6th St.

frontage road

5th St.

Sabine St.

35

700
650
600
550
500
450
400
350
300

FEET

0.5   1   1.5   2
MILES

to creek level. Head south, downstream, along Waller Creek. (You can also wind through the UT campus upstream along Waller Creek using a variety of campus walkways.) Immediately, you'll begin to appreciate the stonework that lends a picturesque, almost medieval look to the Waller Creek Greenbelt. You will also notice that sometimes-parallel paths run on both sides of the trail, especially through Waterloo Park. (Austin was originally known as Waterloo.)

Immediately cross Waller Creek on the first of innumerable bridges. Spur trails connect to the streets above. Pass under 12th Street, the first of many underpasses. Bats are known to live under these bridges.

Buildings and businesses extend directly to the creek's edge. Symphony Square is in one such urban canyon. Here, a portion of the Austin Symphony sometimes plays on a creekside stage. On the far side of the creek, enthusiasts gather on stone outdoor seats to listen.

Waller Creek Greenbelt isn't all about artificial attractions. Look for nature's handiwork too. Willow trees cling to the edge of the stream. Waller Creek has carved wide, whitish stone flats in the creek bed. Look closely at the rock patterns that eons of water and time have worn. Listen for the song of the water as it flows over the rocks in small cascades during times of flow. Unfortunately, the Waller Creek watershed will catch urban trash after a rain, and you will undoubtedly see the results of improperly deposited litter.

Some office buildings have enhanced their landscaping along Waller Creek, adding gardens. Other businesses, especially bars and restaurants, have added patios to overlook the watercourse. Keep in mind that you can incorporate a meal or beverage into your walk.

I couldn't help but wonder what Austin's founders would think about Waller Creek today. Edwin Waller was sent to this area in 1839 to lay out the city and build temporary government headquarters. Waller later became Austin's first mayor. One of his surveyors supposedly named the creek in Waller's honor. The development of downtown and the University of Texas has made Waller Creek a bona fide urban stream. However the Waller Creek Greenbelt makes the most of what the city was left to work with in our day and age.

Leave the creek bed to climb by steps to Eighth Street. Cross the avenue and then pick up the trail again as it curves along Waller Creek. A tunnel passes under Sixth Street and steps also lead up to the street. Many bars and clubs are along this street. The final block of the walk passes along the creek, past stone sculptures through which fountains flow. The trail rises to Fifth Street at 1 mile. The trail continues to Town Lake, where you can connect to the trails around Town Lake, near Waller Beach.

NEARBY ACTIVITIES

Waller Creek courses through downtown Austin, which offers an array of restaurants and entertainment venues.

WALNUT CREEK TRAIL 17

IN BRIEF

Located in far north Austin, this metropolitan park offers not only hiking trails and the usual baseball diamonds and basketball courts, but also the chance to see something not too common in this part of the world: a cricket match.

DESCRIPTION

Purchased by the city in 1964, the park used to be part of a farm owned by the Gracy family. This part of town is close to the environmental region known as the Black Soil Prairie and was probably ideal for crop growth. Abundant picnic tables are located here if you want to make a day of the outing, and plenty of garbage cans keep the area litter free.

This park is rife with trails and side paths, with more landscape than you could probably explore in a single outing. Several creek crossings, depending on the recent rainfall, can either be crossed without getting damp or may require wading in up to your ankles. Prepare accordingly. These crossings and their approaches can be steep and muddy, so allow enough time to avoid being stuck on the trail after dark.

The trail heads south out of the parking lot and soon reaches a T-intersection, where the path widens and offers you the option of going left or right, along the ridge above the Tar Branch of Walnut Creek. Go right. Shortly along the path you'll reach the first of many forks in the trail. At this point, take the right and head through the thick trees ahead. Once through the dense woods, you'll see a chain-link

KEY AT-A-GLANCE INFORMATION

LENGTH: 2 miles

CONFIGURATION: Loop

DIFFICULTY: Easy

SCENERY: Park environment—trees, birds, and dog owners

EXPOSURE: Moderate

TRAFFIC: Moderate

TRAIL SURFACE: Natural stone, gravel, and dirt

HIKING TIME: 1 hour

DRIVING DISTANCE: 13 miles from the state capitol

ACCESS: Daily, 8 a.m.–10 p.m.; no fees or permits

WHEELCHAIR ACCESS: No

MAPS: ci.austin.tx.us/parks/ parkdirectory.htm

FACILITIES: Restrooms, athletic facilities, and swimming pool

CONTACT INFORMATION: (512) 974-6700; ci.austin.tx.us/parks

Directions

The entrance to the park is located on Lamar Boulevard, between Yager and Braker lanes, west off I-35 North, Exit 244.

GPS TRAILHEAD COORDINATES

LATITUDE: : 30° 40' 10.28"
LONGITUDE: 97° 68' 17.50"

fence and maintenance shed on your right. Just past the shed, the trail cuts to the left and crosses the previously mentioned Tar Branch of Walnut Creek.

On the other side of the creek you'll come to another fork in the trail. Again, continue right. Once again, you'll enter some dense woods, and the trail will climb a bit, emerging from the small stand of trees on top of a hill. From this vantage point, you can see the neighborhood to the northwest of the park, and off to the north stand several open grassy meadows and fields—common sights in the Black Soil Prairie region and a contrast to the more common Hill Country ecosystem.

When you reach the third fork, the trail to the right leads out of the park and into a residential area, so take the fork to the left this time and hike along the main branch of Walnut Creek as it flows downstream. A side spur shortly ahead has a steep drop-off. This little trail is very popular with adventurous mountain bikers, but continue following the trail you're on to the southeast.

After trekking roughly a mile, you see a side trail on your right. This is an out-and-back spur. If you want to shorten the hike, remain on the main loop—otherwise turn right and explore the spur. This smaller trail winds down to the creek and is steep in some parts, so be careful and make sure that plenty of light is left in the day when you take on this part of the hike.

When the trail reaches the creek, you'll find a flat, rocky sandbar. Follow the sandbar all the way to the left, and you'll see that the trail continues on the other side. This crossing will be the trickiest of this hike, so take it slow and easy to be on the safe side. Once on the other side, follow the trail as it parallels the tributary system uphill, where you'll be rewarded with the sight of a small, pretty waterfall. After enjoying this hidden gem, turn around and make your way back to the main trail. Though many side trails are in the area and along the hill, this is the big reward for the out-and-back spur.

Once back on the main trail, you'll again cross Walnut Creek and hike along its north side for a while. The terrain alternates between stands of trees and open meadows. Keep your eyes open for deer—does and fawns in the spring and summer, sparring bucks in the fall. You never know what you'll get to see in an area like this. When you reach the four-way intersection, go to the right and head back down to the creek. You'll reach another crossing that is not as difficult as the first. Once on the other side, stay on the trail to the right and continue your southeast heading. As you near the boundary of the park, you'll cross the creek one last time. The incline on the opposite side is steep, so watch your footing as you go.

When you reach the apex of the incline, you'll come to another fork in the path. The right leads toward Lamar Boulevard and out of the park, so take the left. This section of the trail is larger and flatter than most of the trails and shows signs of more traffic than the other sections. As you follow the trail back to the northwest, you'll again find yourself on the ridge overlooking the Tar Branch. When you reach the trail you entered on, take the right and return to your car.

NEARBY ACTIVITIES

The traditional park offers picnicking, ball fields, and basketball courts.

18 WILD BASIN TRAIL

KEY AT-A-GLANCE INFORMATION

LENGTH: 2.5 miles

CONFIGURATION: Loop

DIFFICULTY: Moderate

SCENERY: Creeks, hills, and typical Hill Country vegetation

EXPOSURE: Moderate

TRAFFIC: Heavy–light, depending on time and trails

TRAIL SURFACE: Packed dirt

HIKING TIME: 2 hours

DRIVING DISTANCE: 13 miles from the state capitol

ACCESS: Daily, sunrise–sunset; $3 entrance fee/adult; $2 entrance fee/children ages 5–12 and seniors

WHEELCHAIR ACCESS: No

MAPS: Trail map and interpretive booklet available at entrance or at wildbasin.org

FACILITIES: None

CONTACT INFORMATION: (512) 327-7622; wildbasin.org

GPS TRAILHEAD COORDINATES

LATITUDE: 30° 30' 60.00"
LONGITUDE: 97° 82' 32.50"

IN BRIEF

Wild Basin offers a wide variety of plant life and terrain within its 227 acres. With views of Bee Creek, portions of the Black-Capped Vireo Preserve, and extensive interpretive information, plan to spend the better part of an afternoon on this hike.

DESCRIPTION

The Wild Basin Wilderness Preserve began as the bicentennial project of seven women who were members of the environmental group Now or Never. They originally attempted (unsuccessfully) to lobby the Texas Parks and Wildlife Department to make the area a state park. They were eventually able to acquire money through fund-raising, private donations, and matching grants to purchase the area and set it aside as a safe haven for local plant and wildlife. The area opened to the public in the early 1980s for use as an outdoor classroom and educational area. Note: Pets and bicycles are not allowed.

The hike begins at the large map display near the collection box on the North Holler Trail. The beginning of the hike slopes down at a not-too-steep angle. Along this descent a creek valley is to your left, as well as another ridge to the north of the preserve, which includes part of the Black-Capped Vireo Preserve. Along the ridges farther downstream, houses are starting to creep into the skyline, as is happening in many of the wilder areas in Austin. As you continue west, you'll merge with the Easy Access Loop.

Directions ———————————————→

Entrance is located off Loop 360 South, west of downtown, south of the Austin Lake Bridge.

N
0   0.1   0.2
mile

WILD BASIN
WILDLIFE PRESERVE

North
Access

Environmental
Education Center

South
Access

Arroyo Vista
Loop

Laurel Trail

The Ledge

Triknee Trail

Possum Trail

Falls Trail

Woodland
Trail

Bee Creek

waterfall

Creek Trail

Madrone Trail

North Capital of Texas Hwy.

360

360

Shortly into the hike, you'll reach an area marked "overlook" on the trail map that offers some of the best vistas on this trail, including the creek that feeds Bee Creek. Numerous plaques offer information on the local birdlife that you may encounter. The vegetation begins to thicken beyond this point as the trail descends toward Bee Creek. Though it's not too steep, caution is warranted in some places to ensure safe footing. You'll reach a side trail to the right, but keep going straight and work your way toward Bee Creek along the Triknee and Possum trails.

When you reach the fork in the trail, turn right. This is now the Creek Trail. When you reach the actual creek, you'll have to make the first of two crossings. Ample large stones in the water will allow you to cross without getting wet, as long as you watch your step. The trail continues to follow along the creek and crosses it again about 0.2 miles from the first crossing. An equal distance up the Creek Trail you'll find a waterfall on the left and a bench and outcrop of rock on which to sit to your right. This is a good spot to take a break and enjoy an incredible view.

Once past the waterfall, the trail forks again. To the left, Madrone Trail leads back down the way you just came and eventually joins back with the Creek Trail by the first crossing. Check out an interesting rock staircase and plenty of lush vegetation here. If you aren't too tired by this point, explore this side trail and then follow the Creek Trail back up past the waterfall for a second look. Otherwise, just take the Falls Trail to the right and start working your way back to the trailhead. You'll encounter one side trail on your right as you start the uphill hike. Keep going straight.

When the trail merges with the Easy Access Loop, you can go to the right to check out the interpretive areas that you missed on the way down, or keep going straight to go to the educational center and eventually to your car. Regardless of which side trails you pick, chances are that you won't see it all your first time and you'll want to make another trip to Wild Basin.

Granger
Lake

21

29

Granger

Circleville

95

95

San Gabriel River

79

FM 112

FM 619

Coupland

95

Brushy Creek

FM 973

290

95

FM 1704

Manor

FM 969

Hutto

79

130

130

130

Walter E.
Long Lake

290

35

195

Georgetown

Rabbit Hill

130

Round Rock

35

45

Wells Branch

1

275

AUSTIN

35

183

23

22

Lake
Georgetown

FM 2338

29

FM 1431

20

183

360

1

360

19

183

183A

Cedar Park

Comanche
Peak

FM 718

Colorado Creek

Oak Hill

71

Liberty Hill

29

San Gabriel River

Round Mountain Road

Round
Mountain

Lake Travis

Bee Cave

Barton Creek

71

29

FM 1174

24

71

FM 2238

NORTH
OF AUSTIN

19 BLUFFS OF THE NORTH FORK SAN GABRIEL RIVER

KEY AT-A-GLANCE INFORMATION

LENGTH: 4 miles

CONFIGURATION: Out-and-back

DIFFICULTY: Moderate

SCENERY: Lakeside woods and fields, bluffs

EXPOSURE: Mostly sunny

TRAFFIC: Moderate–busy on weekends

TRAIL SURFACE: Dirt, grass, rocks

HIKING TIME: 2.5 hours

DRIVING DISTANCE: 40 miles from the state capitol

ACCESS: Daily, 6 a.m.–10 p.m.; $4 day-use fee/vehicle with up to six people

WHEELCHAIR ACCESS: No

MAPS: swf-wc.usace.army.mil/ georgetown/images/gtwn%20 images/images/hikingtrailcdw.pdf

FACILITIES: Water, restrooms at trailhead

CONTACT INFORMATION: (512) 930-5253; swf-wc.usace.army.mil/ georgetown

GPS TRAILHEAD COORDINATES

LATITUDE: 30° 69' 67.22"
LONGITUDE: 97° 82' 75.00"

IN BRIEF

This hike traces an old roadbed along the upper embayment of Lake Georgetown, passing bluffs of the North Fork San Gabriel River. It then opens to a flat before reaching more bluffs, where you can look up the river and beyond. From here, adventurous hikers will scramble up to the bluff line or into a nearby hollow.

DESCRIPTION

This hike encompasses part of the San Gabriel River Trail, built by the U.S. Army Corps of Engineers. The trail, also known as the Good Water Hiking Trail, encircles Lake Georgetown and then ties into city trails on its eastern end, making a trek of more than 25 miles around the lake. For this particular walk, leave Tejas Camp and head east on the San Gabriel River Trail. The level walk leads past bluffs on the north side of the North Fork San Gabriel River and along flats to reach bluffs on the south side of Lake Georgetown, where you can overlook the impoundment and the land beyond.

Pick up the San Gabriel River Trail by leaving the parking area and walking toward the low-water bridge over North Fork San

Directions

From Austin, head north on I-35 to Exit 261, Taylor/Burnet, TX 29. Head west on TX 29 to reach Sewards Junction, the intersection of TX 29 and US 183. From here, head north on US 183 and cross over the North Fork San Gabriel River. Just after the crossing, turn right onto TX 3405. Follow 3405 to CR 258. Turn right onto CR 258 to the low-water bridge crossing of the North Fork San Gabriel River. Tejas Camp is on the left just after the bridge. This hike starts on the south side, the Tejas Camp side, of the low-water bridge.

N

0   0.2   0.4
mile

Lake Georgetown

SAWYER PARK

CR 261

milepost 9

San Gabriel River Trail

San Gabriel River Trail

CR 259

Tejas Camp

P

Tower Road

FM 3405

CR 258

CR 258

N. Fork San Gabriel River

1,100			
1,050			
1,000			
950			
900			
850			
800			
750			
700			

FEET

0.5   1   1.5   2

MILES

Gabriel River. Before crossing the bridge, look right for the path and begin following an old roadbed, passing Tejas Camp on your right. The North Fork San Gabriel River flows to your left. At this point, folks can be seen swimming, fishing, or tubing the river into the lake, where the waters are still. This area was historically known as the West End Crossing. It was the fourth upstream river crossing from Georgetown in pre-dam days. This is the only crossing between here and Georgetown that wasn't flooded by the lake. Hayden Hunt and his brothers settled at West End Crossing and built a log cabin, cotton gin, and corn mill. The bluffs across the river from Tejas Camp hold the family cemetery.

Occasional side trails leave left toward the river. At just over 0.5 miles, the aforementioned white and tan, cedar-studded bluffs tower over the river embayment. Along the trail, look for winged elm. This tree with an unusual name often grows in abandoned clearings. Winged elms are easily identified by their corky "wings" running along their branches. The fiberlike inner bark of this tree was made into rope and used to tie cotton bales in the 1800s.

Fields lie to your right. Bluffs rise in the distance. The San Gabriel River Trail descends to a riverside flat, where a wet-weather stream comes in from the right. This streamlet and the entire San Gabriel drainage is part of the Brazos River system, which enters the Gulf of Mexico near Freeport, south of Houston. The North Fork, where you are, meets the South Fork and Middle Fork of San Gabriel River near Georgetown. Step over the streamlet and cross a field broken by a lone live oak. Skirt around a fence at the end of the field to reach a double-track roadbed. Turn left here, staying on level land. Steep bluffs now rise to your right and ahead of you. Reach a stone post and sign indicating that Tejas Camp is 1.8 miles distant.

Keep forward, passing the mouth of the steep-sided and deep Jim Hogg Hollow to your right. This mini-canyon beckons exploration. The San Gabriel River Trail keeps going forward, stepping over the outflow from Jim Hogg Hollow, and begins to ascend a bluff on wooden steps. The path narrows and tunnels beneath thick woods. To your left, views open, looking up the narrow embayment of the North Fork San Gabriel River. Across the water is wide-open cattle country, settled with a few houses. As you keep forward, you'll shortly hit the 9-mile post. This indicates that it is 9 miles from Cedar Breaks Park and the official beginning of the San Gabriel River Trail. The post is a good turnaround point—the trail descends to flats along the river ahead. However, if you are feeling energetic, explore Jim Hogg Hollow or scramble up the bluffs above you before you leave the area. The bluffs flatten out and offer extensive views of the area.

BRUSHY CREEK REGIONAL TRAIL 20

IN BRIEF

This city of Cedar Park hike utilizes yet another expanding greenway of the capitol region. The trail travels along bluff-laden Brushy Creek, meets Brushy Creek Lake, and makes a loop before backtracking over the lake dam, with views aplenty along the way.

DESCRIPTION

The greenways of greater Austin just keep getting better. Brushy Creek Regional Trail is an ambitious project that is slowly but surely expanding. Along the way it connects numerous parks that together provide a recreation corridor—whether you are hiking, fishing, canoeing, rock climbing, or simply getting out for a picnic. The trail is slated to extend 30 miles end to end, stretching from the Highland Lakes in the west to the suburb of Hutto in the east. This particular stretch, located in Williamson County, connects to parks in the city of Cedar Park. Begin your hike at Champion Park, with numerous facilities and a few short trails of its own, and then travel along Brushy Creek, where bluffs overhang the pea gravel track. The trail then rises to cross the dam of Brushy Creek Lake, where you can overlook this 39-acre body of water. The lake is the centerpiece of the second park, aptly

KEY AT-A-GLANCE INFORMATION

LENGTH: 3.16 miles

CONFIGURATION: Balloon loop

DIFFICULTY: Moderate

SCENERY: Creek and lake

EXPOSURE: Partly wooded

TRAFFIC: Heavy on weekends

TRAIL SURFACE: A little concrete, gravel, natural surfaces

HIKING TIME: 2 hours

DRIVING DISTANCE: 21 miles from the state capitol

ACCESS: Daily, 7:30 a.m.–10 p.m.; no fees or permits

WHEELCHAIR ACCESS: Yes

MAPS: wilco.org/portals/0/ mapside3.pdf

FACILITIES: Champion Park has restrooms and picnic areas; Brushy Lake Park has the same, plus kayak rentals and a sand volleyball court.

CONTACT INFORMATION: (512) 260-4283 or (512) 246-2683; parks.wilco.org

Directions

From Exit 250 on I-35 in Round Rock, take Texas Toll 45 west to Parmer Lane, TX 734. Turn right on Parmer Lane, and follow it north 2.3 miles to Brushy Creek Road. Turn right on Brushy Creek Road and follow it 1 mile to Champion Park, passing Brushy Creek Lake Park. Turn right into Champion Park, and the trailhead is on your right.

GPS TRAILHEAD COORDINATES

LATITUDE: 30° 30' 41.80"
LONGITUDE: 97° 45' 30.90"

N

| 0 | 0.1 | 0.2 |

mile

Enjoy this part of the ever-expanding Brushy Creek Regional Trail.

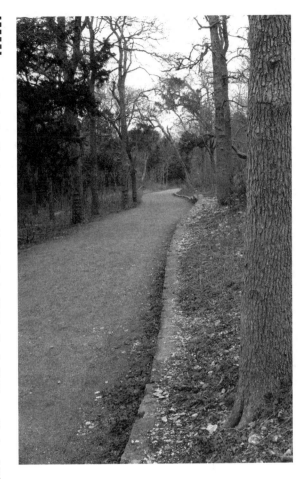

named Brushy Creek Lake Park. This preserve contains not only a loop trail of its own spurring off Brushy Creek Regional Trail but also has kayak rentals in season, a fishing platform, and picnic and play facilities. The regional trail continues beyond this park, but this hike makes a loop and then backtracks across the lake dam and returns to Champion Park. After using this greenway, you will likely push for the trail to be expanded to its full extent, which includes connecting to other paths in the capitol trail network.

The trail is busy with joggers, bicyclists, dog walkers, mothers with strollers, and others, so be prepared to share the path. Champion Park has attractive facilities, from picnic areas under junipers to stonework structures, which you will pass while following a concrete track south toward Brushy Creek. Curve beyond a shaded picnic shelter and children's play area before meeting the Brushy Creek Regional Trail. A short loop path returns to the Champion Park trailhead. Bluffs rise above the creek that babbles beneath vegetation. You turn right, westbound and upstream, on the Brushy Creek Regional Trail with Brushy Creek to your left. The other way heads easterly toward Olsen Meadows Park. The trail bridges Brushy Creek at 0.3 miles. A tributary spills into Brushy Creek just downstream of the bridge. A rock bluff rises beyond the bridge as you work upstream under hardwoods, now on gravel.

At 0.6 miles, the trail switchbacks, climbing to the Brushy Creek Lake Dam. Brushy Creek Lake opens to your left at 0.8 miles. The loop you're about to do is visible below, especially the lakeside part, which tours open terrain, as opposed to the wooded part of the loop that wanders beneath oaks. The Avery Ranch golf course stretches in the distance. The views are continuous as you cross the dam and then curve into Brushy Creek Lake Park at 1.1 miles. Stay left on the Lake

Creek Loop, shortly beginning the circuit portion of the hike. Pass an interior park trail and descend to the impoundment, reaching a kayak rental facility. Sidle alongside still water and look for waterfowl on the lake. At 1.5 miles, a spur trail leads left to a fishing platform and right to a parking area. Keep forward on the loop trail, shortly coming to a shaded lake overlook with picnic tables. Stone bluffs rise from the water.

The loop arcs north along an embayment before reaching a trail junction at 1.7 miles. Here, the Brushy Creek Regional Trail heads west, bridging a small stream, and then tunnels underneath Parmer Lane and on to Brushy Creek Sports Park. Begin circling easterly, passing short nature trails, developed park facilities, and parking on a partly shady track. Complete the loop portion of the hike at 2.1 miles. From here, it is 1.1 miles back to Champion Park.

NEARBY ACTIVITIES

Brushy Creek Lake Park has kayak rentals, a ramp for hand-propelled boats only, picnic facilities, and short nature trails. Champion Park has shaded picnic facilities, its own trails, and playgrounds.

COMANCHE BLUFFS TRAIL 21

IN BRIEF

This hike travels along the shoreline of Granger Lake, an underutilized resource of central Texas. You'll hike through extremely thick forests, which thrive in the fertile soils of the Blackland Prairie. Two historic bridges, which spanned the now-flooded waters of the San Gabriel River, have been moved to the path.

DESCRIPTION

This trail will surprise most central Texans. Simply put, few areas feature such dense woodland. The trail travels through lakeside thickets formed by hardwoods. The path also has open areas that overlook Granger Lake. Damming the San Gabriel River, which crosses the fertile Blackland Prairie, formed Granger Lake. The combination of moist surroundings and rich bottomland are reminiscent of Eastern forests.

Leave the trailhead, immediately descending on the Comanche Bluffs Trail. This is known as the east trailhead. Descend to quickly reach a seemingly out-of-place iron-trestle bridge that far exceeds the dimensions of any normal trail bridge. This is a special bridge, for it is both historic and haunted.

KEY AT-A-GLANCE INFORMATION

LENGTH: 2.4 miles

CONFIGURATION: Out-and-back

DIFFICULTY: Easy

SCENERY: Mostly wooded lakeshore

EXPOSURE: Mostly shady

TRAFFIC: Moderate in summer, very light in colder months

TRAIL SURFACE: Dirt singletrack

HIKING TIME: 2 hours

DRIVING DISTANCE: 44 miles from the state capitol

ACCESS: Daily, 6 a.m.–10 p.m.; closed during draw hunts; $4 day-use fee

WHEELCHAIR ACCESS: No

MAPS: At corps office on way in to trailhead

FACILITIES: Water fountain, restroom at trailhead

CONTACT INFORMATION: (512) 859-2668; swf-wc.usace.army.mil/granger

---

Directions

From Austin, head north on I-35 to Exit 261, Taylor/Burnet, TX 29. Head east on TX 29 for 15.5 miles to reach TX 95 at a T-intersection. Turn right, south on TX 95, and follow it 0.8 miles to Texas Ranch Road 1331, crossing the San Gabriel River. Turn left on 1331, toward Hare, and follow it 4.7 miles to Taylor Park. Turn left into Taylor Park and follow the main road past the entrance station 0.3 miles to the side road, which leads a short distance left to the trailhead.

GPS TRAILHEAD COORDINATES

LATITUDE: 30° 68' 46.11"
LONGITUDE: 97° 35' 21.11"

N

0   0.2   0.4
mile

CR 416

CR 415

FM 1331

entrance
station

Hoxie
Bridge

Trail
Museum

Friendship
Bridge

Granger Lake

CR 496

To primitive-
camp area

U.S. Army Corps
of Engineers
Boundary

FM 1331

To Austin &
35 95

FEET				
700				
650				
600				
550				
500				
450				
400				
350				
300	0.25	0.5	0.75	1	1.2

MILES

The Hoxie Bridge was erected 3.5 miles east of Circleville around 1900, spanning the San Gabriel River where Granger Lake lies today. During the devastating 1921 flood, the Hoxie Bridge was washed 300 yards downstream. In November of that year, a firm was awarded the contract to restore the bridge. A team of convict laborers was sent from Huntsville to aid in the reconstruction. One of the hardened prisoners was a troublemaker. A guard made an example of him, shooting him in the head and hanging him in a nearby tree at the worksite as a grisly reminder to keep the prisoners in line. The bridge was finished and life returned to normal in Circleville. After some time, residents and passersby began to report that the bottomland around the bridge was patrolled by a headless ghost on Friday nights during a full moon. A priest was brought in to pray for the convict's soul and allegedly ended the haunting. In 1979 the bridge was removed from the river before flooding of the lake and was repositioned here by the Army Corps of Engineers. Moving the bridge may have stirred the wrath of the convict ghost, so keep an eye out Friday nights during a full moon.

Ahead, uphill, is the recreation area campground. The Comanche Bluffs Trail veers right and circles the campground. Granger Lake is to your right. Soon you reach the shoreline and pass several cross-trails connecting the lake to the campground, while keeping west in dense hardwoods. The singletrack path works up little hills and down wet-weather drainages.

Climb away from the lake at nearly 1 mile, out to grass and cacti. A final trail from the campground merges with the Comanche Bluffs Trail. Shortly you'll reach the Friendship Bridge. It once spanned Willis Creek, a feeder branch of the San Gabriel River, which now flows into the north arm of Granger Lake.

Bridges like this were important to the development of Williamson County. The rich soils of the Blackland Prairie grew fertile crops, but getting them to market was another matter. The deep stream channels and muddy banks made permanent bridge building difficult until the 1880s. Before then, bridges were low and often swept away by periodic floods. The stronger iron structures with higher abutments made the bridges more reliable. The improved transportation made getting to markets more viable. The same flood of 1921 that ruined the Hoxie Bridge also devastated the Friendship Bridge. The Corps moved this bridge here as well. Today prairie wildflowers grow extensively in this former farmland during April and May.

Leave to the right, away from the Friendship Bridge, shortly spanning a stream on a long boardwalk. Briefly pick up an old roadbed before climbing away from the lake to reach the west trailhead of the Comanche Bluffs Trail at 1.2 miles. Here are a parking area and restrooms. The trail continues 3 more miles beyond to the Fox Bottom Primitive Camp Area. (This camp can only be reached by foot or boat. You must call [512] 859-2668 to register for overnight camping.) The first mile of the trail beyond the west trailhead is fairly easy to follow, but it gets difficult as it winds through thick woods (where driftwood obliterates the trail) and across open prairies (where numerous deer, horse, and foot trails merge and become confusing). Do not continue unless you are an experienced hiker with plenty of daylight to roam. Boardwalks span many of the feeder branches leading into Granger Lake. Parts of the trail are directly along the lake. Otherwise, turn back and enjoy the first portion of the trail a second time. You may want to cut through the campground and check out the Trail Museum, located in the Taylor Park Campground across from campsite #36.

NEARBY ACTIVITIES

Taylor Park offers camping, boating, and fishing in season.

CROCKETT GARDENS AND FALLS 22

IN BRIEF

This is one of the most unsung and best hikes in the Austin–San Antonio area. After tunneling through dense woods, it opens onto tall bluffs overlooking Lake Georgetown. From there, you'll circle around a stream to reach Crockett Gardens and Falls. Here, a crystalline spring emanates from a rock ridge and tumbles over a bluff overgrown with vegetation alongside the falls.

DESCRIPTION

This walk was surprising and a hit from beginning to end and back! The hike encompasses a section of the San Gabriel River Trail, which makes a circuit of Lake Georgetown on U.S. Army Corps of Engineers and city of Georgetown land. The rich cedar woods make for shady hiking, and sheer 100-foot bluffs open up vistas extending the length of Lake Georgetown. Beyond that point, the trail, also known as the Good Water Trail, circles a stream to reach an old homesite and Crockett Gardens and Falls. The springhead flows a short distance to tumble over an unlikely bluff into Lake Georgetown. The rich vegetation around the spring run and falls is attractive and makes a great picnic locale.

Directions ⟶

From Exit 261A on I-35, Lake Georgetown/Andice, take Texas Ranch Road 2338 west. Travel west for 3.3 miles and then turn left onto D.B. Wood Road. Follow D.B. Road west for 2.1 miles, crossing the Lake Georgetown Dam along the way to reach the Cedar Breaks Park entrance station. Take the first left beyond the entrance station and reach the trailhead.

KEY AT-A-GLANCE INFORMATION

LENGTH: 5 miles

CONFIGURATION: Out-and-back

DIFFICULTY: Moderate

SCENERY: Cedar woods, lake bluffs, springs

EXPOSURE: Half sunny, half shady

TRAFFIC: Moderate–busy on weekends

TRAIL SURFACE: Rock, dirt

HIKING TIME: 3.5 hours, including lunch at springs

DRIVING DISTANCE: 32 miles from the state capitol

ACCESS: Daily, 6 a.m.–10 p.m.; $4 day-use fee/vehicle with up to six people

WHEELCHAIR ACCESS: No

MAPS: swf-wc.usace.army.mil/georgetown/images/gtwn%20images/images/hikingtrailcdw.pdf

FACILITIES: Restrooms, water at park picnic area

CONTACT INFORMATION: (512) 930-5253; swf-wc.usace.army.mil/georgetown

GPS TRAILHEAD COORDINATES

LATITUDE: 30° 67' 01.11"
LONGITUDE: 97° 73' 89.17"

Leave the large trailhead on a gravel path extending into cedar woods. At almost 0.5 miles, cross a small, rocky ravine. The gravel has given way to rocks and dirt. Ahead, reach a stone marker. This is Second Booty's Crossing, which in pre-dam days was a route used by travelers up the North Fork San Gabriel River Valley. Originally known as Russell Crossing, this was the second crossing of the North Fork San Gabriel River above Georgetown. The trail of gnarly limestone now makes a bluff line. Here, you can look across the lake at Russell Park. Reach the 1-mile post. Ahead, more views open up, extending the length of the lake. Walk to the bluff's edge—some of the drops are sheer and 100 feet or more down to the alluring blue water.

Continue along the bluff, gaining more views. Pass through an old wire fence and open into a clearing with cacti, rock, and grass. Begin to circle around the embayment of an unnamed stream, passing the 2-mile post. Dip into the sycamore-lined stream, quickly climbing out and to a clearing, where stone relics of an old homestead stand near a cedar-post corral in varied stages of decay. Bisect the corral and reach a trail sign at 2.4 miles. Ahead is Crockett Spring, but turn right here toward the base of the falls. Jump over the streambed below and work around the lake's edge on an old roadbed that now leads into the lake. You'll begin to hear falling water. Across the embayment is Crockett Falls. You can see the narrow stream stair-stepping down a bluff. Lush vegetation lines the falls on its descent.

Return to the main trail and reach the spring run and upper falls. Many a settler has coveted this area. It went through several hands until James Knight operated a flour mill and grew fruits and vegetables in the area, including the first strawberries in Williamson County. Later, R. M. Crockett, who gave the area its name, operated a truck garden. Crockett grew produce and took it to Austin to sell. On the far side of the fence, outside Army Corps of Engineers property, you can see concrete foundations and outlines of buildings, as well as the stone house and corral relics nearby. Large pecan trees shade the spring run and benches. The outflow of the spring is visible near the base of a low rock ridge. The falls from above are quite a sight too. It is easy to see why this is one of the most coveted spots in central Texas.

NEARBY ACTIVITIES

Cedar Breaks Park has a picnic area, campground, and boat landing.

23 OVERLOOK TREK AT GEORGETOWN LAKE

KEY AT-A-GLANCE INFORMATION

LENGTH: 7.2 miles

CONFIGURATION: Out-and-back

DIFFICULTY: Moderate

SCENERY: Lakeside woods and meadows

EXPOSURE: Partly sunny

TRAFFIC: Heavy on weekends

TRAIL SURFACE: Gravel, natural surfaces

HIKING TIME: 3.5 hours

DRIVING DISTANCE: 31 miles from the state capitol

ACCESS: Overlook Park: Daily, 7:30 a.m.–sunset; no fees

WHEELCHAIR ACCESS: Yes, from beginning of trail to nearby fishing platform

MAPS: swf-wc.usace.army.mil/ georgetown/images/gtwn%20 images/images/hikingtrailcdw.pdf

FACILITIES: Overlook Park and Jim Hogg Park have restrooms, water, picnicking, and shelter. Jim Hogg Park also has camping.

CONTACT INFORMATION: (512) 930-5253; swf-wc.usace.army.mil/ georgetown

GPS TRAILHEAD COORDINATES

LATITUDE: 30° 40' 27.10"
LONGITUDE: 97° 43' 25.20"

IN BRIEF

The hike uses the San Gabriel River Trail at Lake Georgetown to connect two developed recreation areas, passing numerous watery vistas along the way, an old ranch site, and an aboriginal Texan village site.

DESCRIPTION

The San Gabriel River Trail, also known as the Good Water Loop, is one of the region's best trail assets. It makes a 26-mile circuit around Lake Georgetown within U.S. Army Corps of Engineers property that envelops the lake. Civilization has reached this reservoir located just west of the now burgeoning suburb of Georgetown. Luckily the lakeshore still exudes a natural aura. This particular hike starts near the reservoir dam, which backs up the North Fork San Gabriel River, and then travels the scenic shoreline, wandering through groves of live oak and cedar separated by grassy clearings, where you can view the main lake as well as intimate coves. Highlights of the hike include these watery vistas, an aboriginal Texan village site, and the stone foundations of a forgotten ranch. Recreation areas on

----

Directions

From Exit 261A on I-35 north of downtown Austin, take Texas Ranch Road 2338, Williams Drive, west for 3.3 miles to D.B. Wood Road and a sign for Cedar Breaks Park. Turn left on D.B. Wood Road and follow it 0.5 miles to the signed right turn for Overlook Park. Follow this road 0.2 miles to dead end at the trailhead. To reach the other end of the trail, take TX 238 5.7 miles to Jim Hogg Road; turn left on Jim Hogg Road to reach the park entrance station. The trail starts on the left just past the entrance station.

N

0   0.2   0.4

mile

FR 2338

Williams Drive

Sedro Trail

Mile 21

entrance station

JIM HOGG PARK

Jim Hogg Road

San Gabriel River Trail

San Gabriel River Trail

FR 2338

Wildwood Drive

Mile 22

foundation

Mile 23

Aboriginal site

Lake Overlook Road

Lake Georgetown

CEDAR BREAKS PARK

Cedar Breaks Road

DB Wood Road

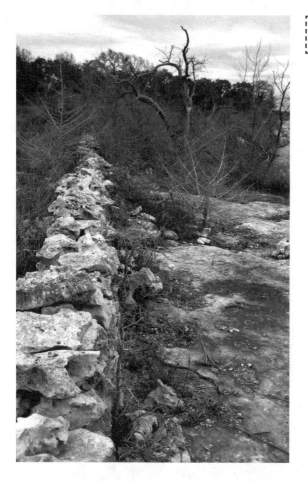

A hand-built stone fence runs near the trail.

both ends of the trail expand your outdoor opportunities. This path is shared with mountain bikers, so listen for their comings and goings.

From the parking area, a concrete walkway descends toward Georgetown Lake. Soon you'll reach a trail junction, with restrooms to your left. Ahead, a path leads to a fishing platform. Turn right here, joining a gravel track, with the trailhead uphill to your right and the lake to your left. This area may be confusing because multiple paths lead from the parking area, but as long as you're heading away from the dam, you'll be fine. Cedar Breaks Park and stone bluffs are clearly visible across the water. Travel an open area and another gravel path splits left toward the lake, but stay right, circling around an embayment. The trail narrows and becomes quite rocky as you pass an old concrete water cistern. Note the sloped rock walls bordering the lake.

Cross the normally dry head of the embayment, passing the mile 23 marker at 0.7 miles. The entire San Gabriel River Trail is marked at one-mile increments. Just ahead you will see the signs indicating the T.H. Godwin aboriginal site, near the water's edge. A rock shelter, midden, and quarry site reveal that aboriginal Texans once lived here. The shelter, ample wood, a spring, and chert made the locale appealing. The aboriginals, with no commutes to jobs and other modern-day distractions, chipped the chert for tools in the shade of the rock shelter. A trail leads down toward the site, but it is now submerged. Continue traveling through a vegetational mosaic of cedar, grass, cacti, brush, and oaks on a rocky track. Pass a "newer" relic at 1.2 miles. Look left for the stone foundation of a ranch house or corral. A long stone fence runs parallel to the lake, which was merely the San Gabriel River when this site was occupied.

Jim Hogg Park, your destination, is visible to the north. Circle a second embayment in suffocating cedars, passing mile marker 22 at 1.7 miles. The scenery changes repeatedly, opening to stony cacti meadows and then piercing dense woods before passing in the shade of live oaks. Another view of Jim Hogg Park and the embayment between you and the park opens at 2.6 miles. Reach the mile 21 marker at 2.7 miles. Enter open terrain on the corps boundary, soon stepping over a trickling branch to meet a bluff just across from your destination. Distant lake views open. Circle around the main embayment. Rock-hop a clear stream at 3.1 miles. Ascend from a wet meadow and then climb a stone bluff. Pass a house on the corps boundary and next join a well-maintained gravel path indicating that you are near the Jim Hogg trailhead. Emerge at Jim Hogg Park at 3.6 miles. The entrance station is visible from here, and parking is available should you choose to make this a one-way endeavor.

NEARBY ACTIVITIES

Jim Hogg Park offers 148 campsites with water and electricity. It is also the western trailhead for this hike. Overlook Park has fishing accesses.

24 RIM ROCK LOOP AT DOESKIN RANCH

KEY AT-A-GLANCE INFORMATION

LENGTH: 3 miles

CONFIGURATION: Loop

DIFFICULTY: Moderate

SCENERY: Riparian creek, prairie, open plateau

EXPOSURE: Mostly sunny

TRAFFIC: Little–moderate

TRAIL SURFACE: Dirt, grass, rocks

HIKING TIME: 1.5 hours

DRIVING DISTANCE: 49 miles from the state capitol

ACCESS: Daily, sunrise–sunset; no fees or permits

WHEELCHAIR ACCESS: None

MAPS: fws.gov/southwest/refuges/texas/balcones/pdfs/doeskin.pdf

FACILITIES: Restroom at trailhead

CONTACT INFORMATION: (512) 339-9432; fws.gov/southwest/refuges/texas/balcones

GPS TRAILHEAD COORDINATES

LATITUDE: 30° 61' 01.11"
LONGITUDE: 98° 08' 15.83"

IN BRIEF

This trail system is a little-known hiking gem. A set of trails has been established in this unit of the Balcones Canyonlands National Wildlife Refuge at the old Doeskin Ranch. This unit of the refuge, northwest of Austin, travels through prime golden-cheeked warbler habitat, first along a creek and next through open grasslands and up to a plateau, where Hill Country views await. A short side hike includes a serene pond.

DESCRIPTION

This little getaway is one of those hikes you want to keep to yourself but can't resist sharing. Leave the trailhead and circle around a feeder branch of Cow Creek. Climb through grassland to reach a plateau where views of Texas Hill Country await. Circle back down, enjoying a bit more creekside canyon scenery before completing your loop.

The golden-cheeked warbler, which lives only in central Texas, is the primary reason for the establishment of the Balcones Canyonlands National Wildlife Preserve, which preserves other species while conserving the warbler habitat. When Spanish explorers named the layers of hills northwest of Austin *Balcones,* they had no idea that their name

----

Directions ──────────────→

From Austin, take US 183 north into the town of Cedar Park. Turn left on Texas Ranch Road 1431 and follow it west for 26 miles to Texas Ranch Road 1174. Turn right and head north on RR 1174, following it for 4.6 miles. Look right for the Doeskin Ranch. A sign will also indicate that this is part of the Balcones Canyonlands National Wildlife Refuge. A short paved path leads down to the main trailhead.

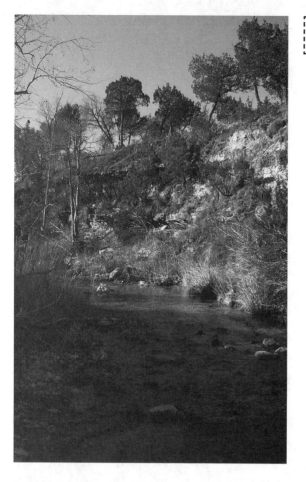

would carry through the ages. But these limestone hills and spring-fed canyons are a treasure worth preserving.

Doeskin Ranch is just one unit of Balcones Canyonlands National Wildlife Refuge. Other units are scattered in the hills south. Start your Doeskin Ranch exploration by taking the Creek Trail past a wooden crib left over from the days when this was a working ranch. Curve past a stone fence, another relic of the past, before working down toward the unnamed feeder branch of Cow Creek. Cypress and sycamore trees line the watercourse. Large boulders lying in the creek have fallen from the limestone walls. The path skirts the divide between creekside woodland and grassland. Follow this perimeter to meet the Rim Rock Trail at just over 0.5 miles. Turn left here, following the roadbed. (The singletrack Rim Rock Trail ahead of you is your return route.) Shortly you'll cross the creek. Stepping-stones have been placed here for easy crossing. A small cascade falls just below the road. Notice the bat box that has been placed in the open land just beyond the stream. The boxes provide critical nesting sites for these insect-eating mammals.

The Rim Rock Trail angles through open land, heading for a draw. Ascend the draw, leaving the roadbed. The singletrack path winds through thick juniper and oak woods to reach a rocky plateau. Look back to gain views from where you came. Briefly walk along the plateau and reach a trail junction at 1.3 miles. Turn left on the Shin Oak Trail, a roadbed. It cuts across the open plateau and then turns right at the junction with the 1.6-mile Indiangrass Trail, which makes a loop of its own that you can use to extend this trek. Amble over the open country with successive junipers emerging from the grasses, rocks, and cacti. The vistas of the adjacent Hill Country are many. Look in the distance and see if you can spot Hickory Pass, the road cut through Tater Hill on Texas Ranch Road 1174, the auto route to Doeskin Ranch. The Shin Oak Trail curves around the edge of the plateau, passing the other end of the Indiangrass Trail to reach the Rim Rock Trail at 1.8 miles. Turn left here, dipping off the plateau on a singletrack path. Many switchbacks ease the descent. The trailhead is easily visible below. The woods give way to grassland, briefly broken by a live oak grove. Keep descending to reach the creek again. Stepping-stones make this crossing easy too. Head upstream, passing a side branch flowing out of the nearby pond. Shortly you'll reach the end of the Rim Rock Trail and turn left, returning to the trailhead at 2.6 miles. Before you leave, however, take the time to walk the nearly half-mile Pond and Prairie Trail, which overlooks a stock pond and the creek. Contemplation benches have been placed along the pathway.

NEARBY ACTIVITIES

Balcones Canyonlands National Wildlife Refuge is made up of many units. Bird-watching, hunting, and hiking are the primary activities on the system.

N

0   7.5   15
miles

SOUTHEAST OF AUSTIN

25 BASTROP STATE PARK LOOP

KEY AT-A-GLANCE INFORMATION

LENGTH: 3.3 miles

CONFIGURATION: Loop

DIFFICULTY: Moderate

SCENERY: Deep pine woods, creek valley, oak forest

EXPOSURE: Mostly shady

TRAFFIC: Moderate

TRAIL SURFACE: Pine needles

HIKING TIME: 2 hours

DRIVING DISTANCE: 35 miles from the state capitol

ACCESS: Entrance fee required

WHEELCHAIR ACCESS: No

MAPS: Online at tpwd.state.tx.us

FACILITIES: Restrooms, picnic areas

CONTACT information: (512) 321-2101; tpwd.state.tx.us

GPS TRAILHEAD COORDINATES

LATITUDE: 30° 11' 14.44"
LONGITUDE: 97° 26' 86.39"

IN BRIEF

This hike loops through the heart of Bastrop State Park. Begin at a vista overlooking the loblolly pine woods that led to this park's creation and travel along Copperas Creek through a deep, shady forest reminiscent of eastern Texas. The moist, intimate stream valleys are also home to the rare Houston toad.

DESCRIPTION

Bastrop State Park is one of Texas's older state parks. It was dedicated in 1937. Land acquisition had been going on for a few years earlier, during the Great Depression. Civilian Conservation Corps (CCC) workers developed the park. The natural reason for its being are the Lost Pines, an isolated pocket of loblolly pines that is mixed with understory species such as oak and yaupon and is separated from similar woods of east Texas by more than 100 miles. At the park's inception, founders didn't realize they were also protecting the greatest concentration of the rare Houston toad, which lives in only a few counties in Texas. The Houston toad is 2–3.5 inches long and varies from light brown to gray or purplish gray, sometimes with green patches. They like deep, sandy soils because they are poor burrowers, but they must burrow into the sand for protection from cold

Directions

From the Austin airport, head east on TX 71 for 25 miles to TX 95 in Bastrop. Turn right and drive north on TX 95 for 0.4 miles to TX 21. Turn right and head east on TX 21 to reach the park, on your right. Pass the park entrance station, then turn left on Park Road 1A and follow it for 1.2 miles to the trailhead, on the right. Start the hike on the Red Trail, near the stone shade shelter.

0   0.15   0.3
mile

N

Lost Pines Trail

Roosevelt's Cutoff

old roadbed

Lost Pines Trail

Park Road 1C

Park Road 1A

Bracken Fern Trace

Scenic Overlook Trail

Post Oak Spur

Copperas Creek Campground

Creekside Campground

Lake Spur

Farkleberry Spur

Pine Warbler Trail

Piney Hill Campground

Deer Run Campground

Park Road 1A

cabin area

BASTROP
STATE PARK

entrance
station

21

150

71

71

700
650
600
550
500
450
400
350
300

FEET

0.5   1   1.5   2   2.5   3   3.3

MILES

weather in winter and hot, dry conditions in summer. Pine-oak woodlands, such as those found here, are ideal for the toad. For breeding they require still or slow-moving waters, such as Copperas Creek, which lies along this trail. Houston toads are active year-round under suitable temperature and moisture conditions. Their diet consists mainly of insects and other invertebrates. The Houston toad population exceeds 2,000 in Bastrop County alone.

This hike through Bastrop State Park starts at the interesting shade shelter, erected by CCC workers on the edge of the Copperas Creek Valley. This round, gazebo-like stone structure beckons you to look inside. Descend from the gazebo by switchbacks on the red-blazed Scenic Overlook Trail into the valley. Avoid short-cutting the switchbacks, as this increases erosion. Enter rich pine woodland. Roll up and down a couple of draws, staying with the red blazes as they moderate the steep hillside grades to meet Bracken Fern Trace. This is the first of many trail junctions. Stay with Scenic Overlook Trail to bridge upper Copperas Creek. Shortly intersect the Lake Spur. Relish the pines shading the path. Reach Farkleberry Spur in a clearing, then span Copperas Creek on a bridge with handrails. Ahead, Scenic Overlook Trail meets Pine Warbler Trail. Shortly, Post Oak Spur leads left.

Despite all the intersections, you've traveled only 1 mile on Scenic Overlook Trail. Keep moving down Copperas Creek, looking right for the brick remains of an old, defunct water fountain. Rock-hop Copperas Creek before intersecting Piney Hill Spur on a small but pretty bluff overlooking Copperas Creek. Soon you'll arrive at the walk-in tent campsites of Copperas Creek Campground. Reach the pavement and walk through the main Copperas Creek Campground, looking for campsite 54. Turn left on the paved road here and take the trail splitting campsites 55 and 56 in a mini-loop. Pay attention here as the trail leaves the mini-loop and comes to a gravel parking area. Veer right here to reach and follow Park Road 1A around a curve.

Ahead at mile 1.7, on the left, is Lost Pines Hiking Trail and a signboard about Houston toads. Take Lost Pines Hiking Trail as it passes a side trail leading to a Boy Scout camping area. If you are thirsty, visit the water fountain at the group camping area. The trail resumes and enters sandy, open ground. Oaks and cedars are more prevalent here. At mile 2.3 turn left at a trail junction onto Roosevelt's Cutoff, staying away from the main loop of Lost Pines Hiking Trail. The path descends into a pine thicket, where pines reflect in dark, pine-stained waters of a dammed trailside pond. Beyond the pond, a few small clearings harbor cacti before coming to yet another junction and the end of Roosevelt's Cutoff. A sign indicates the scenic overlook, your starting point, as almost 0.5 miles distant. Pass through one last swath of rich, dark woods before climbing to reach Park Road 1A and the end of the loop.

NEARBY ACTIVITIES

The park has two good campgrounds, cabins, and picnic areas and is near the historic town of Bastrop. A 13-mile scenic drive connects Bastrop State Park with Buescher State Park to the east.

BUESCHER HIKING TRAIL 26

IN BRIEF

This trail circles through the western end of the Lost Pines, an outlier stand of loblolly pines reminiscent of the piney woods of east Texas. At Buescher State Park, the pinewoods are located on both level land and in deep ravines, adding ups and downs to this loop.

DESCRIPTION

This is an underhiked trail in an underutilized state park. Hikers should consider incorporating other activities—such as camping, swimming, and fishing—into a trip here. Nearby Bastrop State Park gets most of the action in these parts, though Buescher has good scenery as well. Both share a slice of the Lost Pines, a stretch of loblolly pine forest much like that in east Texas. The Buescher Hiking Trail travels exclusively amid the Lost Pines, where yaupon

- -

Directions ————————————→

From the junction of US 183 and TX 71 near the Austin airport, take TX 71 east for 35 miles to TX 95 South/Loop 230, Smithville/Flatonia exit. Get off the divided highway and turn left onto FR 153 (which is not listed on the exit sign off TX 71). Turn left and head north for 0.6 miles to the Buescher State Park entrance. Pass the park entrance, and stay on Park Road 1. After 0.8 miles, you will see the Buescher Hiking Trail trailhead on your right. Do not start here. Instead, drive just a short distance farther and then turn right onto Park Road 1C. Follow Park Road 1C for 1.7 miles to the entrance of the University of Texas Science Park. A parking area is on the left just beyond the entrance to the science park. Pick up the Buescher Hiking Trail as it crosses the road to the science park, heading northeast, the same side as the parking area, and away from the state park entrance.

KEY AT-A-GLANCE INFORMATION

LENGTH: 4.2 miles

CONFIGURATION: Balloon

DIFFICULTY: Moderate

SCENERY: Pinewoods

EXPOSURE: More shade than sun

TRAFFIC: Light–moderate

TRAIL SURFACE: Leaves, pine needles, dirt, some rocks

HIKING TIME: 2.25 hours

DRIVING DISTANCE: 44 miles from the state capitol

ACCESS: Daily, 6 a.m.–10 p.m.; $4 entrance fee/per person over age 13

WHEELCHAIR ACCESS: No

MAPS: tpwd.state.tx.us/ publications

FACILITIES: Water, restroom at picnic area

CONTACT INFORMATION: (512) 237-2241; tpwd.state.tx.us/spdest/ findadest/parks/buescher

GPS TRAILHEAD COORDINATES

LATITUDE: 30° 04' 81.94"
LONGITUDE: 97° 15' 88.61"

N

0   0.1   0.2
mile

To
FR 153

Park Rd. 1C

Raven Road

CR 165

**BUESCHER
STATE PARK**

Buescher Hiking Trail

Park Rd. 1C

P

University Of Texas
Science Park

To
71

700
650
600
550
500
450
400
350
300

FEET

1   2   3   4   4.2

MILES

Loblolly-pine forest

and oaks complement the tall evergreens that reach for the sky. Desiccated ravines break the terrain where the pines grow their richest, and hikers experience some vertical variation.

Pick up the Buescher Hiking Trail as it crosses the Science Center Road. The walking is easy and level amid loblolly pines, live oaks, and red oaks. Copper-colored rocks dot the trail bed. On the way in you may have noticed the elaborate stonework done on park buildings and shelters. The Civilian Conservation Corps (CCC) built these back in the 1930s. The rock slabs were cut from this very same rock. A few buildings of the science center are visible off the path. The singletrack path reaches the loop portion of the hike at 0.4 miles. Turn left here to cross Park Road 1C. A shady mix of woods darkens the path as you curve along a ravine. Shortly dip into the gulch. Notice the forest is richer here—the oaks and pines are bigger. The ravine collects and preserves moisture and helps protect the trees from temperature extremes, enhancing the growing environment.

Span a small ravine on a boardwalk; then climb to level land. The contrast in the two forests is evident. The plateau area is more exposed to the sun's drying influence and is more open. The trees are smaller and somewhat stunted. The walk on level land doesn't last long—the trail begins working into another ravine before reaching a shortcut trail at 1.4 miles. The shortcut leads just over 0.5 miles across the loop. The main path is littered with pine needles as it descends into a bigger ravine, known as Pine Gulch. You may see pools of water in the base of

Pine Gulch or even flowing streams in the cooler months or following rains. Begin cruising down Pine Gulch, a beautiful little valley that exudes a wilderness aura. Before long, the trail dips to the base of the gulch and crosses over the streambed. Climb away from Pine Gulch to cross Park Road 1C at 1.8 miles.

Continue to enjoy the fragrant pinewoods. A nickname for the loblolly pine is rosemary pine for its fragrant and resinous foliage. In other places it is known as bull pine for its giant size. Loblolly pine is the major commercial pine in the Southeastern states. It is extensively cultivated. Its natural range extends from southern New Jersey to Florida and west to Texas. The pines here are at their most westerly range.

Travel over small, undulating hills to reach CR 185, Old Antioch Road, at 2.6 miles. The Buescher Hiking Trail travels alongside a shallow streambed. Parts of the forest open up as you reach an old dirt road at 3.1 miles. To the left is a gated private road. Here the trail splits. Stay left, toward the gated entrance but not through it, as the trail leaving right is the other end of the just over 0.5 miles shortcut. Keep winding through the woods and come across a dammed pond. Reach a final trail junction at 3.8 miles. This is the beginning of the loop portion of the path. Keep forward this time and backtrack nearly 0.5 miles to complete the hike.

NEARBY ACTIVITIES

This state park offers camping and fishing as well as hiking.

LOCKHART STATE PARK TRAIL 27

IN BRIEF

Enjoy the birds and wildlife on this short jaunt around the south side of Lockhart State Park. This is a great walk to take the kids on before heading over to the swimming pool or enjoying a round of golf on the only Texas Parks and Wildlife–run golf course.

DESCRIPTION

When the Great Depression had the nation in a state of despair, young men joined President Franklin D. Roosevelt's CCC with the hope of making a living and maybe a difference. Of the more than 1,400 work camps in the nation, 15 were located in Texas, and they were responsible for a great number of the state-park and forest facilities still in use today. Lockhart State Park is one of those places that benefited from their presence.

Men working for anything from $30 to $40 a month built numerous buildings, roads, and dams across the state. In Lockhart they constructed a swimming pool that utilizes the spring water alongside Plum Creek, in addition to a bridge over the creek that adds to the aesthetic qualities of the park. The park work was complete in 1938, but it wasn't used as a state park until 1948. In that interim period it was leased to a nearby country club.

The trailhead is located near a small bridge and dam of Clear Fork Creek. Here the water trickles at a leisurely pace, and golfers often take a break to wet a fishing line from

----

Directions

To reach the park, go 1 mile south of Lockhart on US 183 to FM 20. Go southwest on FM 20 for 2 miles to Park Road 10; then go 1 mile south on Park Road 10.

KEY AT-A-GLANCE INFORMATION

LENGTH: 0.7 miles

CONFIGURATION: Loop

DIFFICULTY: Easy

SCENERY: Hardwoods

EXPOSURE: Shady

TRAFFIC: Very light

TRAIL SURFACE: Dirt

HIKING TIME: 30 minutes

DRIVING DISTANCE: 35 miles from the state capitol

ACCESS: Daily, 8 a.m.–10 p.m.; $2 entrance fee/person over age 13

WHEELCHAIR ACCESS: No

MAPS: tpwd.state.tx.us/ publications

FACILITIES: Restrooms, vending machines, swimming pool, nine-hole golf course

CONTACT INFORMATION: (512) 398-3479; tpwd.state.tx.us/spdest/ findadest/parks/lockhart

GPS TRAILHEAD COORDINATES

LATITUDE: 29° 84' 89.72"
LONGITUDE: 97° 69' 32.22"

their golf carts. To the right of the creek, you can see the trail leading into the trees under a thick, shady canopy. This little-used trail looks inviting and could very well have inspired Robert Frost's poem "The Road Not Taken," had he lived in Texas instead of New England. Even in the summer a bed of leaves is on the otherwise dirt trail, which is wide enough to allow two or more to walk abreast. The light through the treetops creates shadows that dance on the trail surface. As you start down the trail, Clear Fork Creek can be seen to the left. In the morning, nutria can be seen swimming back and forth in its clear waters, and turtles lounge around all day long. To the right, the dense woods hide foxes, deer, and rabbits, as well as numerous species of songbirds.

About halfway into the hike, you will reach a fence. Turn right and walk beside it for a while. The forested area gives way to grassland that falls victim to the occasional controlled burn, which is sometimes evident, either by charred ground or very new growth. After following the fence for about 200 yards, the trail cuts to the right back into the woods and narrows to allow only one hiker at a time. The trees and ground cover crowd the trail, and the incline gains about 50 feet over the next 0.2 miles.

Songbirds remind hikers of their presence vocally, but they are rarely seen in the thick woods. Fallen trees scattered to the sides of the path show the age of the flora in the park, which has probably never been cultivated. The oaks and cedars have stood undisturbed for centuries. Keep an eye out for spiderwebs crossing the trail. Because the trail sees little use, resident arachnids—some of which grow to a pretty remarkable size—can build some very intricate traps. The thick ground growth also serves as inviting habitat to scorpions, snakes, and tarantulas. Though not as big as the ones seen in the movies or the National Geographic specials, these hairy spiders are big enough that you'll want to avoid them. Chances are that if you do see one, it will be darting or jumping out of your way.

When the trail turns to the right again, it widens back to its original size. This very gentle slope leads back down toward the parking lot, but not before affording you the opportunity to watch cardinals and doves cross the trail above, while lizards and rabbits cross it below. Another 0.3 miles and the trail ends in the parking area, less than 50 yards from where it began.

NEARBY ACTIVITIES

If you have the time and your golf clubs, you can squeeze in a round of golf. You could also head over to the spring-fed swimming hole. Or you could head south to Palmetto State Park to enjoy a hiking trail there, included in this book. If you drive that way, stop in Luling for some of the best barbecue around.

28 LOST PINES HIKING TRAIL

KEY AT-A-GLANCE INFORMATION

LENGTH: 8.1 miles

CONFIGURATION: Loop

DIFFICULTY: Moderate–difficult

SCENERY: Pinewoods, creek bottoms

EXPOSURE: Mostly shady

TRAFFIC: Moderate

TRAIL SURFACE: Pine needles, leaves, dirt, sand

HIKING TIME: 4.75 hours

DRIVING DISTANCE: 35 miles from the state capitol

ACCESS: Daily, 8 a.m.–10 p.m.; $4 entrance fee/per person over age 13

MAPS: At park or at tpwd.state.tx .us/publications

FACILITIES: Water, picnic table, restrooms in day-use area near park pool

CONTACT INFORMATION: (512) 321-2101; tpwd.state.tx.us/spdest/ findadest/parks/bastrop

GPS TRAILHEAD COORDINATES

LATITUDE: 30° 11' 14.44"
LONGITUDE: 97° 26' 86.39"

IN BRIEF

The Lost Pines Hiking Trail is an outstanding path. It offers an attractive, lengthy loop in a wooded setting in which backpacking is a possibility. Forested valleys, mini-gorges, and wood ravines divide pine- and oak-covered hills. The trail is both well marked and well maintained.

DESCRIPTION

The Lost Pines Hiking Trail starts across Park Road 1A from the stone gazebo. Immediately descend into tall loblolly pines—their needles drop onto the understory vegetation and carpet the forest floor a rusty red. The trail bed becomes sandy and the forest opens before reaching Overlook Junction at almost 0.5 miles. Veer left here as the trail bed narrows to a singletrack footpath winding amid small clearings and through scattered pine belts and oak domes.

By now you have noticed the metal rectangular markers nailed to trees at eye level. Their positions indicate the direction the trail travels. At 0.7 miles, cross the Old Road Bed. This former road divides the area. Backcountry camping is allowed beyond this point. However, ground fires are prohibited. The

Directions

From the Austin airport, head east on TX 71 for 25 miles to TX 95 in Bastrop. Turn left and drive north on TX 95 for 0.4 miles to TX 21. Turn right and head east on TX 21 to reach Bastrop State Park. Pass the park entrance station, turn left on Park Road 1A, and follow it for 1.2 miles to the trailhead, on your right. The Lost Pines Hiking Trail starts on the far side of the road from the stone gazebo at the parking area.

Lost Pines Hiking Trail then ascends a hill past an old fence line. The hill is rich with loblolly pines.

Reach County Road 180 at just over 1.5 miles. Cross the dirt road. Ahead, the trail passes over the dam of a pond. Soon pick up a straight, wide roadbed that contrasts with the winding nature of the path so far. The trail shortly leaves the roadbed and melds with the rounded shapes of nature: an old pine log, the bough of a cedar tree, and smooth creek pebbles.

The trail begins to skirt the north edge of a creek valley. The unnamed creek feeds Alum Creek. Views can be had into the creek valley. A multitude of green shades are seen below: bright green pine needles, darker green cedar trees, duller green oak leaves, and lighter yaupon leaves. Their fallen comrades color the ground with varying shades of brown. Drop into the valley, passing an unusual bent oak tree that could be used as a seat, and then reach the unnamed creek at mile 3. The trail crosses the watercourse. This is the first of numerous crossings. These creek crossings are easy except in times of flood, when you shouldn't be on this trail at all. Notice the little bluffs the creek has cut into the hillsides. The Lost Pines Hiking Trail crosses a power-line cut and then returns along the streambed to make a trail junction at mile 3.8. This is known as Buescher Junction. At some point a trail will leave left to connect Bastrop State Park with nearby Buescher State Park.

For now, stay right with the Lost Pines Hiking Trail and cross the creek one last time for good measure. The path climbs and curves back to the northwest, crossing the power-line cut for a second time, and then comes to another pond. This clear pond is fed by a small streamlet. These ponds are good habitat for the Houston toad, with a known realm of nine Texas counties. The toad's best habitat is here at this state park. The 3,000 to 4,000 remaining amphibians are active year-round but burrow to escape extreme heat and cold. They live on insects, such as ants. Keep along the watercourse, heading upstream. Pass another pond shortly before reaching CR 180 at mile 6. Traverse the dirt road and top a hill, dropping into mostly lush woods. Keep an eye out for some of the largest loblolly pines along the trail just before again crossing the Old Road Bed to leave the backcountry camping area of the trail.

Look for a rock outcrop on the trail left just before reaching Roosevelt's Cutoff at mile 7.1. Turn right on a sandy track, heading toward Overlook Junction. The trees stay tall as you reach a pretty pond. Pines ring the coffee-colored water. The woods open up some before reaching Overlook Junction at 7.7 miles. Leave Roosevelt's Cutoff and turn left onto the sandy track and make your way nearly 0.5 miles back to the trailhead, digging deep for that last bit of energy on the final climb.

NEARBY ACTIVITIES

Bastrop State Park has two good campgrounds, cabins, and picnic areas and is near the historic town of Bastrop. A 13-mile scenic drive connects Bastrop State Park with Buescher State Park to the east.

MONUMENT HILL HISTORY AND NATURE WALK

29

IN BRIEF

This hike showcases the site of Texas independence heroes' tomb, a pioneer's house, and brewery, all set on a bluff offering extensive views into the Colorado River Valley. Come on weekends and enjoy guided walks.

DESCRIPTION

Have you heard of the Black Bean Incident? Back when Texas was fighting for independence from Mexico in 1842, a group of militiamen from nearby La Grange went to battle with members of the Mexican army, led by Gen. Adrian Woll, who had captured San Antonio. Woll routed the militia at Salado Creek. A group of Texans crossed into Mexico in retaliation, but most were captured by the Mexican army and forced to march toward Mexico City. Some escaped from the march but were soon recaptured. Following the escape, President Santa Anna ordered every 10th Texan executed. One hundred seventy-six beans were put in a pot, 17 of which were black. Each Texan was ordered to pull a bean. Those who plucked one of the black beans were executed on March 23, 1844.

In 1847 a survivor who plucked a white bean, John Duesenberry, led the retrieval of the executed. The remains, along with those who had battled Woll in 1842 at Salado Creek, were buried in 1848 on what is known as Monument

KEY AT-A-GLANCE INFORMATION

LENGTH: 1.25 miles

CONFIGURATION: Figure eight

DIFFICULTY: Easy

SCENERY: River bluff, sculpted lawn, oak woods

EXPOSURE: Mostly shady

TRAFFIC: Moderate on weekends

TRAIL SURFACE: Wood, rock, gravel, sidewalk

HIKING TIME: 1 hour

DRIVING DISTANCE: 67 miles from the state capitol

ACCESS: Daily, 8 a.m.–5 p.m.; no entrance fee

WHEELCHAIR ACCESS: Yes, on Interpretive Trail

MAPS: tpwd.state.tx.us/publications

FACILITIES: Picnic area, restrooms

CONTACT INFORMATION: (979) 968-5658; tpwd.state.tx.us/spdest/findadest/parks/monument_hill_and_kreische_brewery

Directions

From Austin, take TX 71 east to TX Business 71 near La Grange. Turn right onto TX Business 71 and follow it east 2.2 miles to US 77. Turn right, and head south on US 77 for 1.6 miles to TX Spur 92. Turn right on TX Spur 92 and follow it 0.4 miles to the park, on your right.

GPS TRAILHEAD COORDINATES

LATITUDE: 29° 88' 82.50"
LONGITUDE: 96° 87' 71.94"

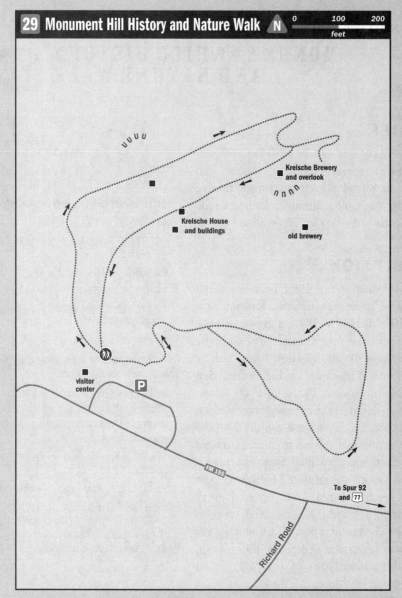

Kreische Brewery
and overlook

Kreische House
and buildings

old brewery

visitor
center

P

FM 155

To Spur 92
and 77

Richard Road

700
650
600
550
500
450
400
350
300

FEET

0.25   0.5   0.75   1   1.25

MILES

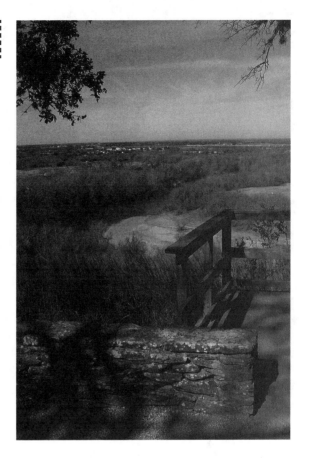

View of the Colorado River

Hill. Later a tomb and monument were built to memorialize those who sacrificed their lives for Texas independence. This state park was established in 1983 after additional lands were acquired, including the home and brewery of Heinrich Kreische, all located on a bluff overlooking the Colorado River Valley and the town of La Grange below.

Leave the visitor center and meander through the well-manicured, oak-studded lawn along the Interpretive Trail with explanatory signage. Shortly reach the monument and internment location of the Texas heroes. On first glance it is hard to believe the grounds were severely neglected before it became a state park. Pass the monument to reach an escarpment overlooking the Colorado River and the town of La Grange. The Kreische house is set back just a bit from the bluff line. Tours of the home are available on some Sundays. Check ahead with the park if you want to join a tour. The Interpretive Trail now heads along the bluff line to reach more stunning vistas looking northward. A long-range telescope allows you to gain closer views.

Turn away from the bluff and come to a side trail to another view. This one looks down into the ruins of Kreische's brewery in a small oak- and cedar-studded valley beside a small spring-fed stream below. You can see the elaborate rockwork by Kreische incorporating the natural slope of the land into the brewing process. Brewery tours are also available on weekends. Return to the main trail and cruise behind the house and outbuildings. Check out the barn, smokehouse, and millstone. You may well wonder how he got any work done with such a fine vista so close at hand. The Interpretive Trail leads back to the visitor center, which has more information inside. Now trace the Nature Trail as it makes a small loop into the upper part of the spring valley. Signposts indicate interesting flora of the landscape. Check with the park rangers for corresponding literature that explains the natural side of this historic spot.

30 PALMETTO STATE PARK LOOP

KEY AT-A-GLANCE INFORMATION

LENGTH: 2.18 miles

CONFIGURATION: Loop

DIFFICULTY: Easy

SCENERY: Riverside riparian woods, swamp

EXPOSURE: Mostly shaded

TRAFFIC: Busy on weekends

TRAIL SURFACE: Compressed gravel

HIKING TIME: 1.5 hours

DRIVING DISTANCE: 58 miles from the state capitol

ACCESS: Daily, 8 a.m.–10 p.m.; $3 entrance fee/person over age 13

WHEELCHAIR ACCESS: Yes

MAPS: tpwd.state.tx.us/ publications

FACILITIES: Restrooms, water, picnicking at trailhead

CONTACT INFORMATION: (830) 672-3266; tpwd.state.tx.us/spdest/ findadest/parks/palmetto

GPS TRAILHEAD COORDINATES

LATITUDE: 29° 35' 23.41"
LONGITUDE: 97° 34' 57.14"

IN BRIEF

This loop traces a revamped trail system at this old-time state park. Travel bluffs along the San Marcos River on a gravel track. Cruise through wooded wetlands, bridging tributaries to reach a swamp forest where the park's namesake plant thrives in impressive concentrations.

DESCRIPTION

This park has been characterized—vegetation-ally speaking—as the place where east meets west. This state park is named after the dwarf palmetto, a ground plant related—as you can guess—to the palm tree. The range of dwarf palmetto is primarily east of Texas throughout the lower Southeast into Florida, though a relic population grows in Oklahoma. On this hike you will see plenty of palmettos. The trek first takes you along the San Marcos River, follow-ing its bends for a good distance, traveling through hardwoods above the banks. The hike then cruises into a marshy area with numerous bridges crossing sloughs. Higher, drier ground harbors mesquite trees, representing the West.

Directions ————————————————————→

From exit 632 on I-10 east of San Antonio and south of Austin, take US 183 south for 2.3 miles to Park Road 11. Follow Park Road 11 for 2 miles to a four-way junction. Keep forward, still on Park Road 11. Shortly pass the park headquarters on your right and pay the entry fee. Then continue over three bridges to turn left 0.8 miles beyond the park headquarters at the sign for the picnic area. Stay with Park Road 11 and follow it to a split. Go left to reach a parking area and stone CCC shelter. Park here. After parking, walk back to the split and then head for the trailer camping area. The trail starts at the beginning of the camping loop by the San Marcos River.

N 0   0.1   0.2

mile

FM 2091

River Trail

big
sycamore
tree

P

iron
bridge

San Marcos River

Park Road 11

Palmetto
Nature Trail

PALMETTO
STATE PARK

To
FM 2091

CR 273

450

400

350

300

250

200

FEET

150

100

50

0

0.5   1   1.5   2   2.18

MILES

Palmetto bushes form a thick tropical understory.

The trek's final distance joins the Palmetto Nature Trail, where you can see palmettos by the hundreds in a swampy setting and also learn about other plants and animals that call this park home. A booklet at the trail's end may lure you to backtrack and do the 0.6-mile nature trail in its entirety.

Palmetto State Park is one of Texas's oldest preserves. Coming in at a mere 270 acres, the park was developed by the CCC in the 1930s. The corps's handiwork can be seen at the trailhead. Here stands a stone picnic shelter overlooking the San Marcos River. The park also offers two camping areas, one of which is at the hike's beginning. Water enthusiasts like to fish, tube, and canoe the San Marcos River. The park also has a 4-acre oxbow lake where you can rent pedal boats and fish. A short nature trail circles the oxbow lake.

Pick up the River Trail heading northeasterly, with the trailer camping area to your right and the San Marcos River to your left. The revamped trail system has a 4-foot-wide pea-gravel bed. Pass behind campsites. User-created paths spur left toward the river below. A shady hardwood forest heavy with hackberry rises over the path. Shortly leave the campground behind. Hikers that have been here before may recognize where the old trail traveled. The reworked trail system was reopened in 2009.

Reach a bend in the river. Bluffs rise across the water. The spring-fed San Marcos River originates 60 miles northwest in the town of San Marcos. This section is one of the last stretches before it joins the Guadalupe River a few miles south, near Gonzales. As you walk along the bluffs, you'll notice that the river in this part of the state is sometimes muddy due to the eroding banks that border it. The San Marcos is subject to flash flooding, evidenced by the numerous dead logs, brush piles, and flotsam high above the river itself.

Travel rich bottoms with tall deciduous trees. Pass a giant double-trunked sycamore at 0.5 miles. The mostly level track makes for an easy hike, allowing you to focus on the scenic surroundings. At 0.8 miles span an intermittent streambed on an iron bridge. Just beyond here a spur path leads right, looping toward the campground. Keep forward, undulating slightly, still along the river. At 1 mile reach the first of two nature trails going right. Stay left unless you want to shortcut your loop. Shortly turn south, aiming for a part of the park that was seldom visited before the new trail system was established. The trail spans often-wet sloughs. Multiple bridges were built to cross these wet areas, separated by drier mesquite patches. At 1.6 miles reach the most southerly part of the hike near the park boundary. The loop turns northwest from here. Palmettos increase in number and you meet the Palmetto Nature Trail at 2 miles. Wander through swampy terrain in thick, almost tropical-looking woods. Emerge onto Park Road 11 at 2.2 miles. Here is a box with interpretive information corresponding with numbered posts. Grab the booklet and backtrack if you want to learn more, returning the booklet after you are done. Otherwise, walk east on Park Road 11 a short distance to reach the parking area.

NEARBY ACTIVITIES

The park also offers camping and fishing. Paddlers can float the San Marcos River, beginning 14 miles upstream at Luling City Park to end here at Palmetto State Park.

WEST
OF AUSTIN

31 BACKBONE RIDGE TRAIL AT LONGHORN CAVERN STATE PARK

KEY AT-A-GLANCE INFORMATION

LENGTH: 1.2 miles

CONFIGURATION: Balloon

DIFFICULTY: Easy–moderate

SCENERY: Cedar, oaks, granite outcrops

EXPOSURE: Open–shady

TRAFFIC: Moderate

TRAIL SURFACE: Gravel, dirt

HIKING TIME: 45 minutes

DRIVING DISTANCE: 64 miles from the state capitol

ACCESS: Daily, sunrise–sunset; closed Christmas Eve and Christmas, as well as during public hunts; no entrance fee; guided tours available for a fee

WHEELCHAIR ACCESS: No

MAPS: longhorncaverns.com/map_trailguide.html

FACILITIES: Restrooms, picnic areas, gift shop, and concession area open later and close earlier than the rest of the park; hours vary by season. Camping and more hiking are available at nearby Inks Lake State Park.

CONTACT INFORMATION: (877) 441-CAVE; longhorncaverns.com

GPS TRAILHEAD COORDINATES

LATITUDE: 30° 68' 43.89"
LONGITUDE: 98° 35' 08.33"

IN BRIEF

Longhorn Cavern State Park, a 650-acre preserve, offers a look at trees and wildlife typically found in the Highland Lakes area. The hike joins the park's two trails as it wanders through cedar stands and passes by and over limestone rocks.

DESCRIPTION

Longhorn Cavern State Park has a lot of history. The caverns, after which the park is named, have seen some colorful characters in their time. Apparently outlaws used it as a hideout in the 1800s. The infamous Sam Bass, who met his end north of Austin in Round Rock, is rumored to have hidden stolen gold here, and local lore suggests that Native Americans held settlers captive here until they were rescued by the Texas Rangers. The nearly 650-acre tract of land was acquired by the state in 1932 and opened as a state park in 1938. Visit the interpretive center to learn more about the cave and the land through which this hike passes.

This is probably one of the easiest trailheads you'll ever have to find. The trail starts right outside the back door of the park office. A sign that reads NATURE TRAIL clearly marks the beginning of the path.

Like many state park trails, the first part of this hike has numbered points of interest that match an interpretive flyer available from the park office. The flyers, however, are limited in number and may not be available, so you may want to print it out online before you

----

Directions

From US 281, north of Marble Falls, take a left on Park Road 4. Longhorn Caverns State Park is on the left.

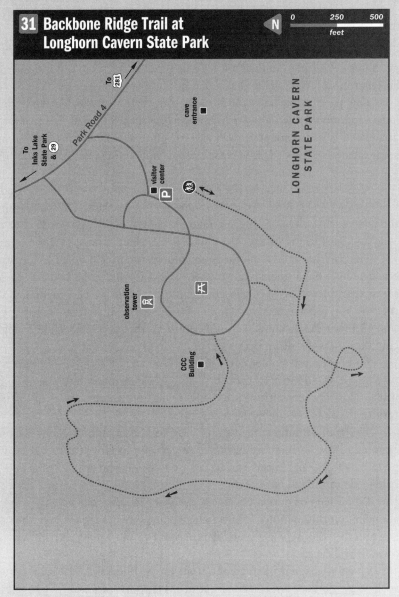

N

0   250   500
feet

To **281**

Park Road 4

To
Inks Lake
State Park
& **29**

cave
entrance

visitor
center

P

observation
tower

CCC
Building

LONGHORN CAVERN
STATE PARK

go. Some of the sites pointed out include types of trees and other flora, as well as an outcrop of limestone used as a den by various animals.

This part of the trail is very easy to traverse—ideal for a family hike with kids—and would even allow for a rugged stroller. The path is made of pressed gravel and is wide enough to walk two or more abreast in most places. Although some shade is provided, it is clear enough in some places to warrant a hat and sunscreen.

After walking for a quarter mile, you'll encounter a fork in the trail, where you'll see a bench. A sign points to more hiking on the left. If you're not up for things to get a little more rugged, take the right fork, which will lead to the park road and back to the office. If you wish to continue hiking, take the left fork.

The trail stays the same for a while longer and includes a couple more numbered points, but it quickly narrows to allow for only one hiker at a time. The surface turns to dirt, which can morph into mud if it has been raining. Shortly up the trail you'll encounter yet another fork. Stay to the left to start the loop portion of this hike. Eventually you'll return to this point along the right fork to complete the extended loop.

Another quarter mile up the trail is yet another fork, with a sign reading 3 MINUTE LOOP pointing to the left. This little loop takes less than 3 minutes to walk and offers very little to see that isn't also on the remainder of the trail. The fork to the right continues the main trail.

The trail is fairly obvious and easy to follow and at times is completely exposed to the sky and free of shade. At certain times of year, flocks of migrating pelicans, ducks, and egrets can be seen overhead; you may even spot a solitary bald eagle in the fall or winter.

Large beds of limestone can be seen on the left, and prickly pear cacti are abundant on this section of the trail. At some points along the hike the cacti stick out into the trail, so watch your step. A spine in the leg makes for a very uncomfortable walk back.

Quiet hikers may be treated to some interesting wildlife along the trail. Black rock squirrels (which are actually a masked color variation of the Eastern fox squirrel) are present, and signs can be seen of both armadillos and wild hogs rooting in the dirt along the trails. Birds that frequent the park, including everything from woodpeckers to the orchard oriole, are numerous.

A little over 0.2 miles from the 3 Minute Loop, the trail becomes extremely narrow and the foliage dense. Again, watch out for the cacti. The trail surface remains unimproved dirt and is lined by wildflowers and cedar trees.

At numerous points from here on, the trail turns to rock and is hard to follow. It would be easy to get turned around on this section of the hike. Be sure to scan all directions for the markers when the trail isn't obvious.

As the trail turns south, you'll wind up on a huge bed of limestone surrounded by cedar and oaks. The trail turns a sharp left here. This is the largest section of rock you'll have been on so far, so you'll know to turn left.

Once past the rock, pick up the trail as it begins to widen again as you head for the park road. At the end of this trail on the left, you will find an old stone building that was built in the 1930s by the Civilian Conservation Corps for use as an office. It's worth a picture. Take the park road to the right from this point to return to the connecting trail.

You'll find the connecting trail less than a quarter of a mile down the road. It is unmarked, but the path is obvious. This will reconnect you to the original trail. Turn left to continue along the previously encountered section, and you will find your way back to the park office. The snack bar will be open, and the iced tea will be cold. If you have time, sign up for the guided tour of the caverns.

NEARBY ACTIVITIES

The park offers guided tours of the caverns regularly. Don't pass up a tour of the unique Longhorn Cavern. Also located nearby is the Canyon of the Eagles Nature Lodge, which offers the Vanishing Texas River Cruise up the Colorado River.

32   FOUR-MILE LOOP TRAIL AT PEDERNALES FALLS STATE PARK

KEY AT-A-GLANCE INFORMATION

LENGTH: 4.8 miles

CONFIGURATION: Balloon

DIFFICULTY: Moderate–difficult

SCENERY: River, wooded plateau

EXPOSURE: Mostly sunny

TRAFFIC: Moderate

TRAIL SURFACE: Dirt, rocks

HIKING TIME: 3 hours

DRIVING DISTANCE: 42 miles from the state capitol

ACCESS: Daily, 8 a.m.–10 p.m.; $5 day-use fee/person over age 13

WHEELCHAIR ACCESS: No

MAPS: At park office or at tpwd.state.tx.us/publications

FACILITIES: Water at trailhead, restrooms at campground

CONTACT INFORMATION: (830) 868-7304; tpwd.state.tx.us/spdest/findadest/parks/pedernales_falls

GPS TRAILHEAD COORDINATES

LATITUDE: 30° 30' 88.06"
LONGITUDE: 98° 24' 66.39"

IN BRIEF

This hike circles around a plateau that is bordered on three sides by the Pedernales River, which you must ford to reach the loop portion of the hike. Once on the plateau, you'll earn views of the surrounding Hill Country. This trail is somewhat difficult to follow, as many old ranch roads spur from the main path.

DESCRIPTION

This balloon hike has an invigorating beginning. Set off on the River Trail and descend to reach the Pedernales River. Here, you must ford the river, which can be quite chilly in winter. Climb away from the river and circle around a high plateau on an old agglomeration of ranch roads that can be challenging to follow. However, you are rewarded with good views of the Pedernales Valley below and the Hill Country through which it courses. Also check out the old homesteader cemetery with simple stone graves.

Leave the Pedernales Falls State Park campground on the River Trail. Pass the campground amphitheater before dropping sharply to the Pedernales River. White blazes painted on trees, stumps, and rocks mark the trail. Get

Directions ⟶

This state park is off US 290 at the Hays–Blanco county line, just west of Henly. It can be accessed from Austin via US 290 and from San Antonio via US 281 to US 290. Once at the county line, take Texas Ranch Road 3232 north for 6.2 miles to the park entrance. From the park entrance station, keep going forward 0.7 miles and turn right into the park campground. The hike starts at the River Trail between campsites #33 and #34.

N

0   0.4   0.8
mile

#34

(Parking is between campsites #33 and #34)

#33

PR 6026

primitive trailhead

park entrance station

Regal Creek

trammel crossing

loop shortcut

4-mile Loop

Pedernales River

PEDERNALES FALLS STATE PARK

Ulrich Road

PR 6026

Pedernales Falls Road

RR 3232

RR 2766

To San Antonio

CR 201

To Austin

FEET

1,100
1,050
1,000
950
900
850
800
750
700

1   2   3   4.8

MILES

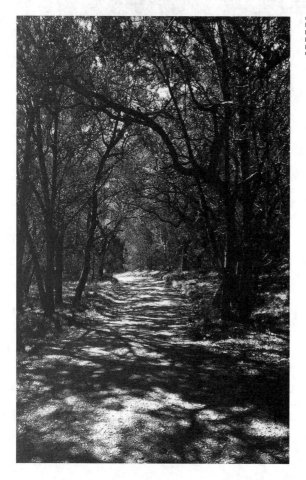

The path as it tunnels through live oak

used to looking for these white blazes—they will help you get around on the far side of the river. For now the path is easy to follow as it bisects a clearing and then enters a hillside of live oaks. Their limbs form a tunnel through which the trail passes. The Pedernales River comes into view, and the green-blue water is appealing to the eye. Cypress trees line the normally clear water. The ford, known as Trammel Crossing, is concrete most of the way across. A long gravel bar and beach lie across the river downstream. Another beach is upstream of the crossing.

In the warmer months, folks will be playing in the water here.

Pick up the wide, gravel path as it climbs away from the Pedernales on the Four-Mile Loop. The gravel gives way once the trail levels off on the plateau. Small meadows and cacti break up the oak and juniper woodlands. The 5,200-acre Pedernales Falls State Park tract was acquired by the state in 1970. At just over 0.5 miles, reach the loop portion of the hike. Stay right here and keep sight of those white blazes in addition to the scenery. You may also notice old stone arrows on the ground. Go against those arrows. Also folks have built cairns (stacks of rock) at trail junctions or where old ranch roads spur off. The trail is level now and becomes rocky in places.

The character of the path changes minute to minute. One trail section will pass through a live oak dome; the next section will be grassy with sporadic juniper. Reach a junction at 1.7 miles. The outer loop portion of the path keeps forward, heading just east of due north, and the loop shortcut leaves to the left. Keep forward on a slight uphill through open juniper lands, passing an old stone fence at 2 miles that obviously once cut through the open land. Stay on the trail to reach a wire fence and the park boundary at 2.3 miles. Turn left here, tracing the fence line. Begin to look left for a short path leading into the woods and the homesteader cemetery. Here, some graves are in a thicket of juniper and live oak. Old wire fences surround some of the sites, while others have piles of rock marking their locations. The names of those interred have been lost to time.

The Four-Mile Loop now makes its biggest climb on the fence line as views open into the ranch country on its far side. Reach a high point and begin to curve west along the fence line. Tremendous views open to the south as the path descends from the high point. Ahead is a wet-weather drainage, heavily wooded with live oak, juniper, and understory brush that can only be described as lush. The trail climbs out of the drainage to level off in a cactus and grass flat at nearly 3 miles. Turn left here, staying with the southbound white blazes.

The level path makes for easy hiking, and at 3.3 miles you'll reach the intersection with the loop shortcut. Stay right here, still on mostly level trailway, drifting in and out of woodland. Complete the loop portion of the hike at 4 miles. Here, backtrack almost 0.5 miles to the river, making the Trammel Crossing one more time. Ascend away from the beautiful Pedernales to complete your hike.

33 HAMILTON POOL TRAIL

KEY AT-A-GLANCE INFORMATION

LENGTH: 1.7 miles

CONFIGURATION: Out-and-back with spur

DIFFICULTY: Easy

SCENERY: Ferns, ash junipers, and hardwoods along the Hamilton Creek and Pedernales River; pool and collapsed limestone grotto

EXPOSURE: Shady

TRAFFIC: Light on trail; busy but limited at pool. Weekends are much busier than weekdays.

TRAIL SURFACE: Dirt, rock, roots

HIKING TIME: 1 hour

DRIVING DISTANCE: 24 miles from the state capitol

ACCESS: Daily, 9 a.m.–6 p.m.; $10 day-use fee/vehicle

WHEELCHAIR ACCESS: No

MAPS: At park

FACILITIES: Picnic tables, restrooms

CONTACT INFORMATION: (512) 854-7275; co.travis.tx.us/tnr/parks

GPS TRAILHEAD COORDINATES

LATITUDE: 30° 34' 12.22"
LONGITUDE: 98° 13' 13.89"

IN BRIEF

This wonderful hike through a unique geological area is more reminiscent of a walk through a canyon in Colorado than the Texas Hill Country.

DESCRIPTION

Like many of the parks and preserves around the Austin area, Hamilton Pool Preserve has a diverse history. Prior to the 19th century, native Tonkawa and Lipan Apaches lived in this area, though cultural remains have been found that date thousands of years earlier.

The preserve is named after Morgan Hamilton, brother to the 10th governor of Texas, Andrew Hamilton. Morgan acquired the property in the 1860s and then sold the land in the 1880s to an immigrant German family named Reimer, who wanted it to graze sheep and cattle. It is rumored that the Reimers' son rediscovered a collapsed grotto, and sometime after that the family opened the area for recreational use. For almost a century the area was subjected to unrestricted use, both by frolickers and livestock, and the land suffered greatly as a result. Five years after the Texas Parks and Wildlife Department declared Hamilton Pool the "most significant natural area in rural Travis County," the county purchased 232 acres from the Reimer family in 1985 and implemented plans to restore it to its original state.

Formed by centuries of water erosion, the canyon provides a natural shelter to a vast

------

Directions

From Exit 229 on I-35, take TX 71 west to Hamilton Pool Road/FM 3238. From Bee Cave on TX 71, drive 13 miles on FM 3238 to the preserve.

N

0   0.1   0.2
mile

Hamilton Pool

waterfall

private property

prairie restoration area

RR 3238

To 71

Hamilton Pool Road

Stagecoach Ranch Road

upland live oak and ash juniper savanna

Pedernales River

RR 3232

West Cave Preserve

FEET

900
850
800
750
700
650
600
550
500

0.25   0.5   0.75   1   1.25   1.5   1.7
MILES

array of birds and wildlife. The rich plant life found here is unusual for this area of Texas. Ferns and ash junipers add an almost prehistoric feel to the valley, compounded by the constantly running water of Hamilton Creek. When visiting the park, please help preserve this unique environment and stay on the trails.

The trail starts where the parking lot ends, leading down into the canyon created by Hamilton Creek. A bulletin board at the trailhead displays pictures of the wildlife and plants found inside the preserve. Numerous bird species and reptiles (including the poisonous Texas coral snake) live here. The coral snake is reclusive and usually spends its time hidden in dead logs, waiting for prey. The preserve is also one of the few places in this part of the state where beavers and porcupines are found. Quiet, early-morning hikers stand the best chance of sighting these creatures.

About 400 feet into the hike is a bench where you can sit and watch the traffic as it comes and goes to the pool, the most popular attraction of the preserve. The trail is steep at times, and it can be interesting to watch people carrying their ice chests to and from the area. Continue down the trail until you reach a T-intersection in the path, where you'll find two portable toilets, garbage and recycling bins, and a directional sign. The pool is on a spur trail to the right, less than 0.1 mile distant, but you'll want to save that until last, so turn left toward the Pedernales River.

The trail parallels Hamilton Creek, which creates a soothing sound as you hike. Many of the trees here are relatively young, though some older trees and the remnants of others can be seen in the form of fallen trunks, logs, and stumps. You'll come to an old dead stump 0.2 miles into the trail, on your right, where you'll see a new tree growing right up through it. Many of the hardwoods here are mesquite, cedar, and oak.

Immediately ahead on the trail, two large boulders lean on each other to form an arch over the trail under which taller hikers will have to duck. Take a moment to study the surface of the rocks, and you'll notice shells embedded in them. Heed a sign here that reminds hikers to remain on the trail to avoid damaging the fragile ecosystem.

Occasional spur trails along the hike include a fork 0.3 miles into the trail that leads down to the creek. At most points, stakes and twine mark the boundaries within which hikers should stay. Where no such markers exist, stay on the trail. Gradually the trail climbs but never too steeply, and eventually it winds up about 20 to 30 feet above the creek. As it continues toward the Pedernales, cliff faces become larger along the left side of the trail. Ferns drape the rocks in numerous places, and caves perforate their surface.

At nearly 0.5 miles into the trail, a stand of junipers creates a natural tunnel of foliage. Keep a sharp eye out for birds crossing the path. They could be golden-cheeked warblers, which are known to nest in the park. At just over 0.5 miles, a roped-off scenic overlook affords a view down into the canyon. The water is incredibly clear, due in large part to the numerous small rapids in the stream, and the prospect of seeing fish and snapping turtles (and the occasional beaver) is good. Continue on to the junction of the Pedernales and Hamilton Creek, 0.8 miles from the trailhead.

Once at the Pedernales, two benches made from cedar posts let hikers rest and enjoy the view. The river is very wide here, and the view is breathtaking. When the river is low, numerous sandbars appear; you can wade out and work your toes in the silt and sand of the river. Numerous fish can be seen, and some of them are quite large. These are gar, and they are quite abundant in this stretch of the Pedernales, all the way down to Pedernales Falls State Park. Keep an eye out for great blue herons and egrets wading along the banks. If you brought a snack, this a good place to enjoy it. When you're ready, turn around and start back down the trail.

When you reach the intersection leading back to the parking lot, continue straight to the pool. The sounds of people playing in the waters ahead will precede your arrival. You'll pass between two large boulders just past the toilets, and at 1.5 miles into the hike, you'll see the clear waters of Hamilton Pool, partially shaded by the large outcrop of the collapsed limestone grotto. A small bridge over the creek leads to the pool, but continue up into the grotto itself for now.

The trail leads up into the large, open cave and hugs the inside wall. Almost as soon as you are under its ceiling, a large piece of rock appears, requiring a tight squeeze through the area it's in. A large metal staircase leads down about 20 feet and overlooks the pool. Watch your step because the stairs are always very slippery.

The small birds you see flying around in the cave are cliff swallows. They make their nests out of mud and hang them like cliff dwellings on the rock wall.

Just as you're exiting the grotto–cave, note a large deposit of lime on the right. Covered in moss, this formation adds the exclamation point to the prehistoric feel of this place. When you're back on the beach, take your shoes off and go for a swim. The water is surprisingly transparent, and fish that get trapped in the pool when the creek is low can be seen circling the banks, looking for a way out. To return to the parking lot, simply cross the bridge, turn right back on the main trail, and head back to the intersection. Climb back up the left fork to find your car.

Note: Entrance is limited to 75 vehicles at a time, and once that limit is reached, no one else is let in until someone leaves. Plan to arrive early because no waiting places are nearby. Pets are not allowed, and camping and fishing are also prohibited.

34   INKS LAKE STATE PARK TRAIL

KEY AT-A-GLANCE INFORMATION

LENGTH: 3.6 miles

CONFIGURATION: Balloon

DIFFICULTY: Moderate

SCENERY: Hills, lake, wildlife

EXPOSURE: Shady, with a few open spaces

TRAFFIC: Light

TRAIL SURFACE: Dirt and rock

HIKING TIME: 2 hours

DRIVING DISTANCE: 67 miles from the state capitol

ACCESS: Daily, 8 a.m.–10 p.m.; $5 entrance fee/person over age 13

WHEELCHAIR ACCESS: No

MAPS: tpwd.state.tx.us/ publications

FACILITIES: Restrooms, showers, picnic tables, and camping. Park store sells refreshments and supplies and rents canoes.

CONTACT INFORMATION: (512) 793-2223; tpwd.state.tx.us/spdest/ findadest/parks/inks

GPS TRAILHEAD COORDINATES

LATITUDE: 30° 74' 99.17"
LONGITUDE: 98° 35' 53.61"

IN BRIEF

Located in the Highland Lakes chain west of Austin, this moderately challenging hike passes through granite hills and wraps around portions of Inks Lake's shoreline. Abundant wildlife and few hikers make this a real gem.

DESCRIPTION

Hiking at Inks Lake State Park seems to be a secondary activity, despite a good trail system. A large sign designates the trailhead and includes a map of the trails available. This hike is composed of a combination of two of them. The third trail leads to the park's primitive camping area and is similar in flora and fauna to this hike.

The trails are color coded and marked accordingly along the trail. The beginning trail's color is green. Following the green markers, begin walking south. The trail starts out wide and easy, with the shade beginning immediately. While you're hiking, you'll encounter slight inclines along the trail, but only a couple of them are steep.

About 0.2 miles into the hike, after you've walked up a slight rise, look directly out in front of you. On a hill in the distance, you'll notice a local anachronism: a castle sitting atop one of the neighboring hills. Although this is actually a resort and hotel, it certainly is a striking landmark of central Texas. This is definitely another reason to bring binoculars on this hike.

Directions ———————————————→

From US 281 in Marble Falls, turn left on Park Road 4 and follow it until you reach the entrance to Inks Lake State Park.

However, the main reason to bring field glasses remains the wildlife. The nature of the foliage along the trail is ideal for attracting fauna. White-tailed deer bed down underneath cedar and oak trees right next to the trail, and an early-morning hiker has a good chance of catching the deer while they are still sleeping. Cottontail rabbits are frequently encountered as well.

Near the same point where the castle is visible, the trail forks to the right. The right fork climbs a limestone hill and then leads back to the improved campsites or dead-ends on the lakefront. Stay to the left to remain on the main trail, which follows the lake farther down the path.

The trail continues through the trees and forks again 0.3 miles from the trailhead. Another sign indicates your current location on the trail. Don't rely only on these maps because they are a little harder to decipher than the park map. The left fork is the Pecan Flats Trail; it leads to the primitive campgrounds. Stay to the right.

You'll climb a small bed of limestone shortly past the fork. A little farther down the trail, you'll see a stone structure through the trees. This is the base of the bridge on the park road. A small wooden bridge is also on the trail for foot traffic.

From here the trail opens up, and the lake appears on the right. This area of the lake is known as Stumpy Hollow and is popular with the bass boats as well as bank anglers. Anglers of all ages try their luck for everything from catfish to crawfish.

While hiking along this part of the trail, the odds of spotting wading birds such as blue heron and snowy egret are excellent. Between the months of November and March, you might even spot a bald eagle—they nest farther up the Colorado River during the winter.

As you continue to hike, the trail leaves the lake and heads up a hill on more limestone. The peak of this hill, at 962 feet, is actually lower than the trailhead, which is 992 feet above sea level. Keep a keen eye peeled for the trail markers because no dirt or footprints are here to follow. The markings are green dots of paint rather than arrows. Watch the ground ahead to see more than one marker at a time.

Just before the peak, the trail is again marked with a sign. Although no map is here, arrows point the way. The right leads through more stone hill, and plenty more is to the left about 0.75 miles ahead. Take the left fork.

When you reach the next fork, take the left one again. The trail to the right loops back on itself around the hill and heads back to the park, offering little more variety. The left trail crosses the park road and leads back into some thicker land. Shortly after crossing the road, the trail forks again. This time go to the right.

Although no benches are along this hike, plenty of large rocks are available on which to rest. A large group of such rocks is located just past the fork. As you continue on the trail, the markers turn blue and are mainly plastic surveyor's tape in the trees. The trail remains fairly obvious and isn't hard to follow. This section is another loop that circles over two small hills.

One of the most obvious landmarks here is a large power line that you'll pass under twice. When you pass under it the second time, you're about two-thirds through this loop. As you start heading back toward the road, you'll come across yet another fork. The trail to the right is marked in red and is an alternate route to the Pecan Flats campground. Stay to the left and complete the loop back to the park road. Cross the road and follow the trail back to the parking lot, retracing your steps back through Stumpy Hollow.

NEARBY ACTIVITIES

If you have some time, you might want to rent a kayak or canoe at the park store and explore the coves of Inks Lake. The park also offers picnicking, camping, and a nine-hole golf course.

35 JOHNSON SETTLEMENT TRAIL

KEY AT-A-GLANCE INFORMATION

LENGTH: 1 mile

CONFIGURATION: Loop

DIFFICULTY: Easy

SCENERY: Historic buildings and longhorn cattle

EXPOSURE: Sunny

TRAFFIC: Moderate–heavy

TRAIL SURFACE: Dirt

HIKING TIME: 20 minutes to walk the trail, but allow more time to explore the settlement

DRIVING DISTANCE: 51 miles from the state capitol

ACCESS: Daily, 9 a.m.–sunset; closed Thanksgiving, Christmas, and New Year's Day; donations accepted; check Web site for hours and fees for tours of buildings

WHEELCHAIR ACCESS: Yes

MAPS: nps.gov/lyjo

FACILITIES: Restrooms at the visitor center; dining and shopping in Johnson City

CONTACT INFORMATION: (830) 868-7128 ext. 244; nps.gov/lyjo

GPS TRAILHEAD COORDINATES

LATITUDE: 30° 27' 49.44"
LONGITUDE: 98° 41' 23.61"

IN BRIEF

This is an easy trail that offers a great look at the people who worked the frontiers of the Texas Hill Country, complete with exhibits and artifacts.

DESCRIPTION

The seeds of Johnson City were planted in the 1850s when President Lyndon B. Johnson's grandfather, Sam Ealy Johnson Sr., settled with his brother Tom in a one-room cabin on 320 acres of prime Texas land. The cabin and additional structures eventually became the headquarters for their cattle-driving business, which started a year after the Civil War ended. The brothers drove their cattle north to market from the Hill Country, where the demand and the prices for beef were high.

Business was initially very good, so they bought an additional 640 acres to expand their operation. Nestled between the Pedernales and Blanco Rivers, their location was ideal for grazing. The cattle market eventually collapsed, and the brothers ended their partnership in 1871. They left Blanco County, selling their interest in the land to Sam's nephew, James Polk (J.P.) Johnson, after whom Johnson City is named. Many buildings J.P. constructed still exist, including a barn and a cooler house to go with the original cabin. The trail begins across the street from the visitor center. Signs here ask that visitors refrain from smoking along the trail and remind them

----

Directions ————————————➤

From Austin, take US 290 West to US 281 North, and from San Antonio, start on US 281 North. When you reach Johnson City, just follow the signs to the downtown area that point out the park.

not to climb into the corrals with the temperamental longhorns. The path is wide and easy to traverse, and parents with strollers should have little problem rolling along the packed-dirt trail. After crossing a wooden bridge, the trail meanders along the edge of an open field where wildflowers bloom in the spring and early summer. A few old live oaks stand along the trail as well.

You'll reach the interpretive center, which resembles an old ranch house, 0.3 miles from the trailhead. Numerous rocking chairs are on the porch, and a huge oak tree is in front. The ample shade of this area encourages visitors to sit down, relax for a while, and try to imagine life in a simpler time. A breezeway is between the restrooms and water fountain.

The self-guided tour inside the center is wheelchair accessible and includes information and artifacts from the early days of the frontier pioneers. One of the highlights of the museum is an actual dialogue composed of correspondence by J.P. Johnson and his fiancée, which has been recorded and plays back for visitors to hear. You can spend an easy hour in here taking in the exhibits.

Past the interpretive center (as you walk through the breezeway), a second bridge leads into the actual settlement area. To the left of the trail is the cedar-fenced corral that contains the longhorns, and another sign cautions visitors to stay on this side of it. An old covered wagon is on the right.

The trail continues toward the original cabin built by Sam and Tom Johnson. The addition of the east room does little to add to the small quarters. The rustic cabin has stood for about 150 years and offers a glimpse into a lifestyle that has long since been forgotten.

A German immigrant named John Bruckner purchased part of the ranch after the brothers ended their business relationship. He is responsible for building the next structure. The cut-stone barn was constructed in 1884. J.P. built the next barn in 1875, along with a two-story frame house that burned down in 1918.

The final structures are a windmill and water tank, as well as a cooling house built by J.P.'s son-in-law N.T. Stubbs. After having taken enough time to investigate the settlement, you can follow the trail around through the grassland, stopping at a bench located under another oak to watch the birds and animals in the field late in the afternoon. The trail joins a fence and turns to the right. Follow this trail back to the beginning of the loop, where you'll turn left to return to the visitor center.

NEARBY ACTIVITIES

Located across the street from the visitor center is LBJ's childhood home. The former president lived here from age 5 throughout his childhood, until he married at age 26. The home has been restored to its 1920s state and is open for tours to the public.

This area is only part of the Lyndon Johnson National Historical Park. The Ranch, located 14 miles west of town, offers a nature trail (included in this book) and a guided bus tour of the president's home.

THE LOOP AT ENCHANTED ROCK

IN BRIEF

Enchanted Rock, arguably the most notable landmark in the central part of the state, is the centerpiece of this loop hike, which encircles the pink-granite mountains that arise from the Texas Hill Country. The breathtaking view from the top of Enchanted Rock extends 360 degrees. Other features along this hike include more vistas, a pond, a canyon, and backcountry campsites. Be prepared to visit during off times, as nice weekends can be so crowded that park entry is cut off.

DESCRIPTION

We'll admit it—Enchanted Rock State Natural Area is outside the distance parameters of this guidebook, but the scenery here is just too good to pass up. Step for step, this is one of the most scenic hikes in central Texas.

Start on the Loop Trail, traveling through open terrain, where views of the surrounding pink-granite mountains and boulder fields are far-reaching and amazing. You will pass a side trail to a vista before reaching a backcountry campsite. You'll enjoy a water feature, Moss Lake, which makes an excellent front stage for the sheer granite monoliths behind it. Next,

KEY AT-A-GLANCE INFORMATION

LENGTH: 4.1 miles

CONFIGURATION: Loop

DIFFICULTY: Moderate–difficult

SCENERY: Open-faced granite mountain, broken woods, canyon walls

EXPOSURE: Almost all sunny

TRAFFIC: Very heavy on weekends

TRAIL SURFACE: Granite slab, pea gravel, dirt, rocks

HIKING TIME: 2.75 hours

DRIVING DISTANCE: 97 miles from the state capitol

ACCESS: Daily, 8 a.m.–10 p.m.; closed during public hunts; $6 day-use fee/person over age 13

WHEELCHAIR ACCESS: No

MAPS: tpwd.state.tx.us/ publications

FACILITIES: Restrooms and water at picnic area and campground

CONTACT INFORMATION: (830) 685-3636; tpwd.state.tx.us/spdest/ findadest/parks/enchanted_rock

Directions

From the Gillespie County Courthouse in downtown Fredericksburg, take Main Street west for 0.3 miles to reach Milam Street/Texas Ranch Road 965. Turn right on Milam Street/RR 965, and follow it for 17 miles to reach Enchanted Rock State Natural Area. Keep forward beyond the park entrance station, crossing Sandy Creek. Turn left at the T-intersection and park toward campground sites #4–#34. The hike starts on the Loop Trail at the far side of an auto turnaround near campsite #22.

GPS TRAILHEAD COORDINATES

LATITUDE: 30° 49' 85.83"
LONGITUDE: 98° 81' 70.56"

travel up Echo Canyon, where the twin towers of Little Rock and Enchanted Rock squeeze the trail. Finally ascend the open granite face of Enchanted Rock, where vistas open up in all directions.

The rewards are big, but so are the crowds. If you are coming to Enchanted Rock on a weekend, be aware that the park often fills its 260-car capacity by 10 a.m. After this time, automobiles will not be allowed into the park until 4 or 5 p.m., if at all, so plan ahead. You might want to call before you come. I suggest overnighting at the campground on the weekend of your visit. The campground reservation number is (512) 389-8900. Better yet, come during the week. Avoid this park completely on holidays and during spring break.

Start the hike on the Loop Trail by passing around a metal gate onto a wide pea-gravel path. The terrain is wide open, broken only by smaller tree stands. A boulder field is in the distance. Spur trails head toward any and all rock formations. Rock climbing is popular here. The domes of Little Rock and Enchanted Rock stand to your right.

Begin to walk among cabin-size boulders, which are strewn about as if they were building blocks tossed by a child. The huge granite slabs beneath your feet will simply amaze you. At slightly more than 0.5 miles, look for a side trail that leads right to an odd standing rock with a hole eroded clear through it—a keyhole of sorts.

Keep in open country, circling around Little Rock, which is little only in comparison to the larger Enchanted Rock. Reach a side trail at 1 mile leading left to a 360-degree vista. You can see other rock formations, among other sights, to the north toward Llano.

Ahead, a trail leads left to Walnut Springs Camping Area. This site is for backpackers, but it does have a restroom. Many red oaks are scattered over the landscape. Leave the Loop Trail at 1.5 miles and then turn right onto the Echo Canyon Trail, soon passing over the dam of Moss Lake. Live oaks offer a shady lakeside resting spot for hikers. The lake and mountains make for a picturesque setting. You can see the sheer granite domes and the boulders that have fallen from the domes over time; in addition, you may see specks of humanity climbing various bluffs and rocks of the domes.

Keep going, heading toward Enchanted Rock, now on a less obvious trail over granite swales. A path leads left for Moss Lake Primitive Camping Area, another backcountry campsite.

Keep straight in this confusing area, aiming for the gap between Enchanted Rock and Little Rock, as an unnamed trail leads left around the north side of Enchanted Rock. You will enter Echo Canyon near a primitive bathroom and then reach a signboard showing climbing routes and other information. Keep going up Echo Canyon, directly up the rocky drainage amid huge fallen boulders. After passing over a high point, you'll then dip onto a sheer granite slab at 3 miles at a sign that indicates the Echo Canyon Trail. You can see others scaling the open face of nothing but rock.

Begin angling directly up Enchanted Rock on the Summit Trail. Stay on the hard ground and avoid the few and unusual weather islands, where vegetation struggles for life as a bit of soil has found a home in a crack or indentation in the hard rock. On hot summer days the sun heats the granite so much that it groans as it cools down after expanding from the heat.

Reach the top of Enchanted Rock and have a look around. Other visitors will be relaxing and taking in the views, which are plentiful and expand in every direction. The actual highest point is on the rock's northwest side. Look down onto Moss Lake and the main park area below—you'll see what resembles a world of toy cars, buildings, and people. The landscape of central Texas stretches off for miles in all directions.

Backtrack on the Summit Trail, descending all the way to a feeder branch of Sandy Creek before taking a few steps past a viewing telescope near a gazebo. You are at the far end of the day-use parking area. Follow the paved road toward the southwest end of the campground and complete your loop.

NEARBY ACTIVITIES

This state park offers hiking, picnicking, rock climbing, and walk-in tent camping.

LYNDON B. JOHNSON RANCH TRAIL 37

IN BRIEF

This great family hike has historical overtones, wildlife, and interpretive signs. Plenty of rest areas, water fountains, and wide trails make this an easy trip for hikers of all ages. Highlights include a working farm frozen in the 19th century.

DESCRIPTION

The peace and serenity of the Lyndon B. Johnson State and National Historical Ranch offer a stark contrast to the tumultuous time in which he served as president. His ranch house located just on the other side of the Pedernales River was the location of many a lawn chair Cabinet meeting when the tribulations of the presidency would follow him to the quiet of his home. Often referred to as the Texas White House, LBJ succeeded in setting up shop where he was comfortable working, and his staff would fly in to his private airstrip to catch up to him.

LBJ and his wife donated this park, along with the ranch that is accessible only by a bus tour, to the nation—a gift to the people and land of which they were so fond. The ranch house contains many of the gifts they received while in office.

The trail begins in a large field of wildflowers by the visitor center. The wide path

KEY AT-A-GLANCE INFORMATION

LENGTH: 1.1 miles

CONFIGURATION: Balloon with out-and-back spur

DIFFICULTY: Easy

SCENERY: Wildlife pens, working farm, hardwoods

EXPOSURE: Mostly shady

TRAFFIC: Busy on weekends; lighter during the week and in the mornings

TRAIL SURFACE: Packed dirt

HIKING TIME: 45 minutes

DRIVING DISTANCE: 65 miles from the state capitol

ACCESS: Daily, 8 a.m.–sunset; no entrance fee

WHEELCHAIR ACCESS: Yes

MAPS: At park office or at tpwd.state.tx.us/publications

FACILITIES: Restrooms, gift shop, vending machines

CONTACT INFORMATION: (830) 644-2252; tpwd.state.tx.us/spdest/findadest/parks/lyndon_b_johnson

Directions

Take US 290 West out of Austin to junction with US 281 North. Take US 281 North to Johnson City and turn left on US 281 West. The park is located 14 miles west of Johnson City on the right. Park in the main parking lot and obtain a map from the park office. The trail begins on the north side of the visitor center and is clearly marked with a large sign.

GPS TRAILHEAD COORDINATES

LATITUDE: 30° 23' 94.44"
LONGITUDE: 98° 62' 80.83"

N

0   250   500
feet

Hodges Ranch Road

Ranch Road 1

290

Pedernales River

Ranch Road 1

wildlife park

Living Historical Farm

Park Road 52

wildflowers

visitor center

P

P

Park Road 52

290

1,600
1,550
1,500
1,450
1,400
1,350
1,300
1,250
1,200

FEET

0.25   0.5   0.75   1   1.1

MILES

meanders to the northwest toward a stand of trees. Located 0.1 mile into the hike is a slightly larger-than-life statue of Johnson, who was born and raised in nearby Johnson City. His actual ranch, which has been turned into a national historic park, is just on the other side of the Pedernales River.

As the path continues, you'll reach a fork about 0.2 miles into the trail. Stay to the right. You'll see the wildlife pens down the fork to the left. Resist the urge to go look at the deer now, as you'll finish the hike returning along this fork.

Just past the fork, you'll cross a wooden bridge over a nameless perennial stream. The trees are dense here and provide ample shade on a warm afternoon. Signs denote some of the different trees along the path, including hackberry, mesquite, and cedar. Occasional plaques provide information about local wildlife along the trail as well.

At 0.3 miles the trail forks again. Stay to the right, which loops out a little way and leads to the Hill Country Woody Plant Exhibit and Rest Area. A billboard contains even more information on the local flora and provides a good place to rest weary little hikers who may have to take more steps to keep up with their older companions.

The trail turns back into the main trail after the rest area and leads to the working historical farm almost 0.5 miles into the hike. This is the first of two main highlights along the trail. Open the gate and step back more than 100 years into the past. Forever frozen in the late 19th century, the farmers here go about their daily chores in period costumes and are more than happy to pose for photos. Chickens, turkeys, and other animals wander around the farmyard, and roosters crow for attention all morning long. A large barn and farmhouse make up the structures here, and visitors are free to examine them more closely at their leisure. Just like the period it preserves, there is no rush around here.

Once you've checked out the farm, return to the trail, where it once again forks. The fork to the right leads to a playground area and picnic tables. Unless you plan on taking a break, continue to the left. You'll go through another gate, back into the perennial creek bottom area and the accompanying hardwoods. You'll reach another fork with a bridge to the left. Take the right fork to head to the Pedernales River overlook, passing up another fork to the right, unless you need to use the restrooms at the end of this spur.

Along the trail on the left, which follows the creek bed, you'll find an information plaque on one of the least-heralded animals in Texas: the nutria. A relative of the beaver, this large rodent can be seen on most of the state's rivers and golf course water hazards. They are responsible for most of the holes you'll find dug along trails in the Hill Country.

Just over 0.5 miles into the hike you'll walk under a bridge for the ranch road, and more water will be evident in the creek bed, which feeds the Pedernales. The overlook is 0.7 miles into the trail. Here you'll find a great view of what, at times, is a wide and strong river. This is the end of the spur and has another plaque with information on the river's bird and fish life.

After you've walked back under the road, look for a fork to the right. A small stone stair crosses the creek bed. This path rejoins the main trail just on the other side of the bridge you passed on the way to the overlook.

You'll begin to see the fence of the wildlife pens on the right, and small spurs in the trail allow you to walk up to the high fence for a closer look. On the other side you'll find longhorn cattle and white-tailed deer. The cattle are usually lying in the tall grass in the heat of the day, but the behemoths are easy to spot. The deer can generally be seen poking their heads around the trees for a look at the hikers.

When the trail turns to the right, you'll see a water tank on the far end of the pen. Deer are also found here most of the time, and some will even approach the fence, looking for a handout from the passersby. Caution is advised with the friendly deer because they are still wild animals and can spook easily.

Turn to the left at the next fork and then right at the next one. One final fork to the left will take you back to the visitor center. Here you can go inside and sign up for the bus tour to Johnson Ranch on the other side of the river; here the former president and his wife are buried in the family's private cemetery beneath the live oaks.

SANDY CREEK HIKE 38

IN BRIEF

This hike at Enchanted Rock State Natural Area is often overlooked by the more popular trek to the top of Enchanted Rock. It is certainly less busy as it travels along clear Sandy Creek, past Frog Pond, and then through the pink-granite mountains that make the Enchanted Rock area so beautiful. The trail is a little hard to follow in places as it loops back around to Sandy Creek.

DESCRIPTION

This hike avoids the throngs that can be heading up Enchanted Rock yet enjoys much of the same scenery. Cruise along the valley of Sandy Creek, crossing over to reach Frog Pond. From here, take Turkey Pass Trail, cutting between Enchanted Rock and Turkey Peak, where granite walls rise on both sides of the trail. Work through a smaller wooded canyon nearing Buzzard's Roost (Buzzard's Roost and Turkey Peak are both rock-scrambling destinations). Return to your destination along the open, pretty Sandy Creek.

The heavy use at Enchanted Rock has resulted in many illegal bootleg trails running

KEY AT-A-GLANCE INFORMATION

LENGTH: 3 miles

CONFIGURATION: Loop

DIFFICULTY: Moderate–difficult

SCENERY: Creek bed, granite mountains

EXPOSURE: Mostly open

TRAFFIC: Moderate–busy

TRAIL SURFACE: Dirt, gravel, rock

HIKING TIME: 2 hours

DRIVING DISTANCE: 97 miles from the state capitol

ACCESS: Daily, 8 a.m.–10 p.m.; closed during public hunts; $6 day-use fee/person over age 13

WHEELCHAIR ACCESS: No

MAPS: tpwd.state.tx.us/ publications

FACILITIES: Restrooms and water at trailhead

CONTACT INFORMATION: (830) 685-3636; tpwd.state.tx.us/spdest/ findadest/parks/enchanted_rock

----

Directions _____⟶

From the Gillespie County Courthouse in downtown Fredericksburg, take Main Street west for 0.3 miles to reach Milam Street/Texas Ranch Road 965. Turn right on Milam Street/RR 965 and follow it for 17 miles to reach Enchanted Rock State Natural Area. Keep forward beyond the park entrance station, crossing Sandy Creek. Turn right at the T-intersection and park. The hike starts near the gazebo and restrooms. However, do not take the Summit Trail. Instead, head for the low-water concrete footbridge crossing Sandy Creek.

GPS TRAILHEAD COORDINATES

LATITUDE: 30° 49' 85.83"
LONGITUDE: 98° 81' 70.56"

N

0   0.2   0.4

mile

Buzzard's Roost
Primitive Campground

compost toilet

RR 965

Loop Trail

Buzzard's Roost

Sandy Creek

Freshman
Mountain

Turkey Peak

Turkey Pass Trail

Frog Pond

Enchanted Rock
(1825')

Summit Trail

park headquarters

To
Fredericksburg

RR 965

maintenance building

Loop Trail

Moss Lake
Primitive Campground

Echo Canyon Trail

compost toilet

Little Rock

Sandy Creek

P

Moss Lake

Walnut Springs
Primitive Campground

compost toilet

Loop Trail

ENCHANTED ROCK
STATE PARK

2,000
1,900
1,800
1,700
1,600
1,500
1,400
1,300
1,200

FEET

0.5   1   1.5   2   2.5   3

MILES

Rock slab between hills near Sandy Creek

just about everywhere. The legal trails, which are better to follow, are marked with low wooden posts inscribed with an arrow and a white plastic diamond. Get used to looking for this sign—certain sections of the hike are hard to follow.

If you are coming to Enchanted Rock on a weekend, be aware that the park often fills its 260-car capacity by 10 a.m. After this time, automobiles will not be allowed into the park until 4 or 5 p.m., if at all, so plan ahead. You might want to call before you come. I suggest overnighting at the campground on the weekend of your visit. The campground reservation number is (512) 389-8900. Better yet, come during the week. Avoid this park completely on holidays and during spring break.

From the northeast end of the day-use parking area, near the restrooms and the gazebo, head away from the throngs heading up Enchanted Rock on the Summit Trail. Instead, walk past the bathrooms for the low-water concrete footbridge spanning Sandy Creek and heading toward the park office. Cross Sandy Creek on the bridge and then turn left, passing through a small picnic area. You are now on the right track, heading downstream in the floodplain of Sandy Creek, which is to your left.

Trail signs indicate the way as you shortly travel under a cathedral of shade-providing hardwoods. The walking is easy. Reach a group picnic pavilion beside Sandy Creek at just over 0.5 miles. Turn left here on the Turkey Pass Trail, rock-hopping the stream, which flows in clear braids over a grainy, tan bed. Frog Pond appears just over the hill from Sandy Creek. Walk along the pond's edge before reaching a junction. Stay right on the Turkey Pass Trail, heading for the gap between Turkey Peak to the right and Enchanted Rock to the left. This is one place where multiple paths spur off, especially toward Turkey Peak, which hikers often climb. The mammoth stature of Enchanted Rock towers to your left.

Reach the gap and keep forward. The trail travels over slabs of granite, making for a wide-open panorama. Freshman Mountain stands in the distance to your right. Broken pieces of granite, in all shapes and sizes, lie at the base of Enchanted Rock. Gravity is obviously doing its work. Drift down through oak woods to reach a trail junction at just over a mile. The Turkey Pass Trail ends here. Turn right onto an unnamed trail, immediately crossing a wet-weather drainage. Keep downstream, parallel to the drainage, before climbing over a hill and dipping into the drainage again. Look for the trail signs. The trail briefly follows the bottom of the drainage before leaving left to join the Loop Trail at 1.6 miles. Buzzard's Roost, a prominent rock formation popular for climbing and scrambling, is dead ahead.

Turn right on the wider, easier-to-follow Loop Trail. It travels amid boulder fields and other pink-granite features between Freshman Mountain to your right and Buzzard's Roost. This area beckons exploration. Descend to cross Sandy Creek. Just ahead the trail leading to Buzzard's Roost Primitive Camping Area leaves to the left. You, however, continue upstream along open Sandy Creek, where gravel bars and many rock formations enhance the stream shed. Views open of Turkey Peak, then of Enchanted Rock up high.

Return to the group picnic shelter at 2.4 miles. This ends the loop portion of your hike. Keep forward along Sandy Creek and backtrack a little more than 0.5 miles to the trailhead.

NEARBY ACTIVITIES

This state park offers hiking, picnicking, rock climbing, and walk-in tent camping.

WOLF MOUNTAIN TRAIL

IN BRIEF

This trail explores the high country of Pedernales Falls State Park. Good views await, as do creeks, a spring, and even a homesite. This rustic swath of the Hill Country offers a true sense of remoteness. For those inclined, the Wolf Mountain Trail also has a backcountry campsite, which can extend your adventure. A side trip to the Pedernales River adds even more beauty.

DESCRIPTION

This is a solid day hike in the Hill Country. This trail is great to hike after a rain-bearing front has blown through, filling the Pedernales River and its tributaries and clearing the skies for far-reaching views. The path ventures across several stream sheds, the last of which has a spring and homesite nearby. Ascend Wolf Mountain to take in vistas of the land beyond and the Pedernales River below.

The Wolf Mountain Trail descends from the parking area into juniper woods to reach a roadbed used only by park personnel. Veer right here, descending past a feeder branch of Regal Creek. A small cascade falls here in times of flow. Climb away, shortly noticing the signs that mark the path in half-mile increments.

KEY AT-A-GLANCE INFORMATION

LENGTH: 7.4 miles

CONFIGURATION: Balloon

DIFFICULTY: Difficult

SCENERY: Mountainside oak–juniper woods, creek valleys

EXPOSURE: Mostly sunny

TRAFFIC: Moderate

TRAIL SURFACE: Dirt, rocks

HIKING TIME: 4.5 hours

DRIVING DISTANCE: 42 miles from the state capitol

ACCESS: Daily, 8 a.m.–10 p.m.; $5 day-use fee/person over age 13

WHEELCHAIR ACCESS: No

MAPS: At park office or at tpwd.state.tx.us/publications

FACILITIES: Water at trailhead, restrooms at park office and near backcountry camping area on trail

CONTACT INFORMATION: (830) 868-7304; tpwd.state.tx.us/spdest/findadest/parks/pedernales_falls

Directions

This state park is off US 290 at the Hays-Blanco county line, just west of Henly. It can be accessed from Austin via US 290 and from San Antonio via US 281 to US 290. Once at the county line, take Texas Ranch Road 3232 north for 6.2 miles to the park entrance. From the park entrance station keep forward 0.2 miles and turn right at the sign for primitive camping and reach the trailhead.

GPS TRAILHEAD COORDINATES

LATITUDE: 30° 30' 57.22"
LONGITUDE: 98° 25' 82.78"

N

0   0.25   0.5
mile

maintenance
building

Park Road 6026

trammel
crossing

4-mile
Loop

Twin Falls

P

Regal Creek

Wolf Mountain Trail

Pedernales River

PEDERNALES FALLS
STATE PARK

Divide
Mountain

Bee Creek

Mescal Creek

Wolf
Mountain

Tobacco Creek

Tobacco
Mountain

Jones
Spring

homesite

High
Point

Long
Mountain

Twin
Butes

Lone
Mountain

Mount
Butler

Park Road 6026

Ranch Road 2766

CR 201

CR 201

To
Johnson City

Ranch Road 3232

To Austin,
San Antonio,
& 290

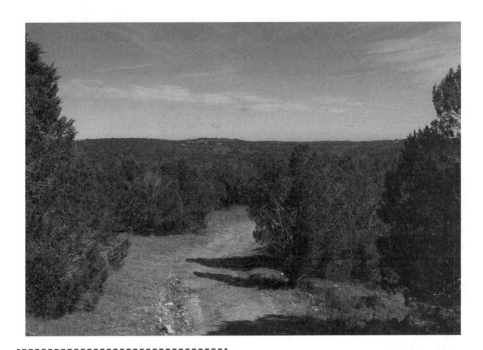

Hill Country near Wolf Mountain

Oak-and-juniper woodland dominates the landscape, which is broken by rough grasses and rocks aplenty. Gray skeletons of long-dead trees litter the landscape. Curve into the Bee Creek watershed, reaching Bee Creek at 1 mile. Ascend away from Bee Creek, passing a high point at 1.5 miles. Wolf Mountain is visible ahead on the downgrade from the high point.

Reach Mescal Creek at 1.8 miles. Climb a bit; then reach a trail junction. Here, a path leading left heads toward the primitive backcountry camping area for overnight visitors. This is also a way to access the Pedernales River. The area below the river bluffs is especially scenic; however, no camping is allowed below the bluffs. Day hikers continue forward to reach another junction and the loop portion of the hike. Keep straight here, shortly passing a primitive backcountry privy. The woodland thickens in spots. Dip down to Tobacco Creek at 2.6 miles. This creek dries up earlier than the other creeks. Pass a grassy meadow just after the 3-mile mark. Ahead, at 3.3 miles, is Jones Spring on a side trail to the left. The spring is set in a creek bed. When the stream is flowing, the water falls in a series of cascades. Look for ferns growing on the north bank of this creek bed.

Ahead on the Wolf Mountain Trail are the rock walls of an old homesite. Undoubtedly the homesteaders decided to build here because of the close proximity to Jones Spring. The trail narrows to a singletrack path beyond the homesite as it twice bisects an old stone fence. While you are walking, contemplate all the hard labor that went into building that fence. Keep ascending along a normally dry streambed amid a thicket of live oaks, deciduous oaks, and junipers.

Turn away from the streambed you have been following just before the 4-mile marker. Ascend a rock slope with a more arid look to it. A real sense of remoteness falls over the land here. The narrow path, ascent, and multitude of rocks make the hiking slower than on the old roadbed. Reach a trail junction at mile 4.6. Veer right here, joining an old roadbed. The trail leading left heads to the park boundary and Blanco CR 201. Shortly ahead is another trail junction. Veer right here, although either way takes you around the peak of Wolf Mountain. The right, or east, side has better vistas. The vistas quickly open up, and you can look out far in the Pedernales Valley and beyond. Ahead, you can occasionally see the unmistakable green-blue color of the river itself. At mile 5.2, meet the trail that came around the west side of the mountain. Descend, looking left for a narrow side trail that leads uphill to a wooden viewing platform.

Reach another junction at mile 5.4. You have been here before. Turn left, backtracking now, passing the backcountry camping area, Mescal Creek, and Bee Creek, returning to the trailhead at 7.4 miles.

NEARBY ACTIVITIES

Pedernales Falls State Park has camping, fishing, mountain biking, river swimming, and tubing.

San Antonio (Hikes 40-51)

N

0 4 8

miles

Bulverde

Cibolo Creek

FM 1863

46

10

Leon Creek

Salado Creek

Timberwood Park

281

FM 1535

46

1604

Bracken

42

211

Black Hill

Helotes

48 Wetmore

35

1604

40
41
45

16

47

Leon Creek

Leon Valley

281

Alamo Heights

Converse

410

1604

10

421

10 90

San Antonio

FM 1515

FM 1957

151

410

90

13

Lackland AFB

13

35 536

51

410

90

Macdona

Medio Creek

Von Ormy

Mitchell Lake

281

Southton

181

Calaveras Lake

37

Braunig Lake

Elmendorf

35

1604

49

Medina River

Earle

San Antonio River

1604

16

SAN ANTONIO

40 BLUFF SPURS OVERLOOKS

KEY AT-A-GLANCE INFORMATION

LENGTH: 4.6 miles

CONFIGURATION: Balloon loop with spurs

DIFFICULTY: Moderate–difficult

SCENERY: Open and wooded hill country

EXPOSURE: Partly open

TRAFFIC: Busy on nice days

TRAIL SURFACE: Natural surfaces

HIKING TIME: 2.5 hours

DRIVING DISTANCE: 25 miles from the Alamo

ACCESS: Friday–Monday, 7 a.m.– 10 p.m.; $6/person over age 13

WHEELCHAIR ACCESS: No

MAPS: tpwd.state.tx.us/ publications

FACILITIES: Restrooms, water, picnicking, visitor center at trailhead

CONTACT INFORMATION: (210) 688-9055; tpwd.state.tx.us/spdest/ findadest/parks/government_ canyon

GPS TRAILHEAD COORDINATES

LATITUDE: 29° 32' 55.00"
LONGITUDE: 98° 45' 54.20"

IN BRIEF

If you like a hilly, challenging trek enhanced with rewarding vistas, this hike is for you. Government Canyon State Natural Area is the setting for this circuit that travels the nexus of hill and grassland before climbing into wooded prominences broken with outcrops that avail extensive vistas.

DESCRIPTION

Greater San Antonio continues to spread outward, taxing the Edwards Aquifer, which is the primary water source for the city. The state of Texas established Government Canyon State Natural Area to help recharge the aquifer, literally flowing through cracks, sinkholes, and caves into large caverns that comprise the aquifer. More than 7,500 of the 8,000-plus acres of the state natural area are in the aquifer's recharge zone. The two other aquifer zones are known as the drainage zone—where water is actually captured at the surface and then flows into the recharge zone—and the discharge zone, where water flows out of the aquifer as natural springs or is removed through man-made wells.

The springs of Government Canyon drew farmers and ranchers here. Later, San Antonio spread, and land speculators saw a development for 80,000 residents. However, scientists

---

Directions ———————————→

From the intersection of Loop 1604 and Shaenfield Road, northwest of downtown San Antonio and south of Braun Road, take Shaenfield Road west for 1.6 miles to a traffic light. Continue forward through the traffic light, as Shaenfield Road becomes Galm Road. Keep west on Galm Road and follow it 1.9 miles to the entrance on your right. Once in the park, drive to the visitor center. The trails begin there.

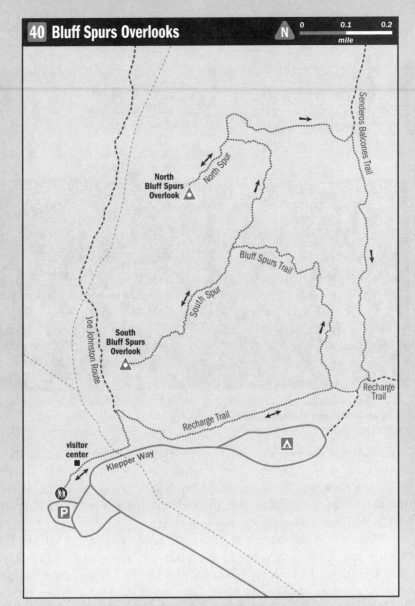

N   0   0.1   0.2
mile

Senderos Balcones Trail

North Spur

North
Bluff Spurs
Overlook

Bluff Spurs Trail

South Spur

South
Bluff Spurs
Overlook

Joe Johnston Route

Recharge Trail

Recharge Trail

visitor
center

Klepper Way

P

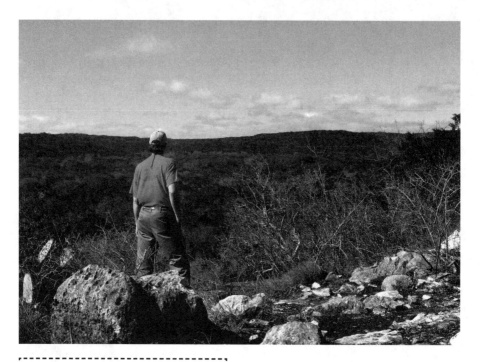

A view from the South Bluff Spurs Overlook

and residents came to understand the importance of Government Canyon in relation to the aquifer. The area was purchased by the state in 1992. Government Canyon is now open for exploration. This hike travels an important fault line of the recharge zone and then climbs to overlooks that will add to your appreciation of the aboveground beauty and the aquifer below.

From the visitor center take the trail leaving easterly beyond the Edwards Aquifer information display to cross Government Canyon on a road bridge. Immediately reach the backcountry trailhead. Turn left here, traveling up the Joe Johnston Route to intersect the Recharge Trail after a quarter mile. Turn right on the Recharge Trail, walking easterly along the fault line that separates the Balcones Escarpment, which you are about to climb, and the flatlands to your south. Meander through a mix of meadow, cacti, rock, and cedar. At 0.4 miles, a closed path leads right to Klepper Way. Stay left with the Recharge Trail, intersecting the hiker-only Bluff Spurs Trail at 0.8 miles. Turn left here, ascending north on a narrow track. The landscape continually changes from open rock to cacti gardens to juniper thickets. The irregular climb leads to a trail junction at 1.3 miles. Turn left, southbound on the South Spur. Descend before reaching the edge of Government Canyon and a rock outcrop at 1.7 miles. The state natural area visitor center and attendant buildings are visible below. Views extend well beyond to your south and west. Backtrack to reach the Bluff Spurs Trail at 2.1 miles. Travel north on a single-track path in a mix of sun and shade. At 2.4 miles, reach the North Spur. Stay left, southbound through crowded tree thickets, to reach another rock opening and vista at 2.6 miles. The park headquarters is visible again, but you can see farther into the Hill Country this time, as this overlook is 100 feet higher than the South Bluff Spurs Overlook. Rejoin the main loop at 2.8 miles, traveling easterly to meet the Sendero Balcones Trail, a multiuse path, at 3.1 miles. Walk southbound on this ridgeline track. Watch your feet, as the path is very stony. Views open to your south on the descent, another reason to take it easy on this trail. Pass an old stock fence just before meeting the Recharge Trail at 3.6 miles. Trace the old roadbed westerly, shortly passing a side trail leaving left to the park campground. Complete the loop portion of your hike at 3.8 miles. Begin backtracking on the Recharge Trail, returning to the visitor center and parking area at 4.6 miles.

NEARBY ACTIVITIES

Government Canyon State Natural Area offers drive-up tent and RV camping, backcountry camping, and picnic facilities.

41 CHULA VISTA LOOP

i KEY AT-A-GLANCE INFORMATION

LENGTH: 7.2 miles

CONFIGURATION: Loop

DIFFICULTY: Difficult

SCENERY: Open and wooded hill country, canyon

EXPOSURE: Partly open

TRAFFIC: Semi-busy on nice days

TRAIL SURFACE: Natural surfaces

HIKING TIME: 3.8 hours

DRIVING DISTANCE: 25 miles from the Alamo

ACCESS: Friday–Monday, 7 a.m.–10 p.m.; $6/person over age 13

WHEELCHAIR ACCESS: No

MAPS: tpwd.state.tx.us/publications

FACILITIES: Restrooms, water, picnicking, visitor center at trailhead

CONTACT INFORMATION: (210) 688-9055; tpwd.state.tx.us/spdest/findadest/parks/government_canyon

GPS TRAILHEAD COORDINATES

LATITUDE: 29° 32' 55.00"
LONGITUDE: 98° 45' 54.20"

IN BRIEF

This long loop explores the highs and lows of Government Canyon State Natural Area. Head up Wildcat Canyon, enjoying riparian scenery, before climbing into lofty terrain. Join a ridgeline where far-reaching views await from rock outcrops. Two named vistas highlight the overlook possibilities.

DESCRIPTION

The Balcones Escarpment rises from the lower end of Government Canyon, providing the vertical variation for this hike. Leave the visitor center, which is worth a visit, and travel up Government Canyon, passing relic structures from ranchland days. Leave Government Canyon to enter Wildcat Canyon, exploring riparian bottom where vegetation grows lush around stony washes that flow during big rains. Travel the streambed and crisscross braids of the wash as well as side canyons flowing into Wildcat Canyon. The vegetation becomes noticeably smaller upon ascent into the high country, where you will pass the High Lonesome Windmill. The loop hike joins the most easterly trail in the park while exceeding the 1,300-foot elevation mark, wandering a knobby ridge. Rocky openings provide broad outlooks where you can see near and far, including downtown San

----

Directions ————————————————→

From the intersection of Loop 1604 and Shaenfield Road, northwest of downtown San Antonio and south of Braun Road, take Shaenfield Road west for 1.6 miles to a traffic light. Continue forward through the traffic light, as Shaenfield Road becomes Galm Road. Keep west on Galm Road and follow it 1.9 miles to the entrance on your right. Once in the park, drive to the visitor center. The trails begin there.

N

0   0.25   0.5

mile

Twin Oaks Trail

Senderos Balcones Trail

High Lonesome Windmill

△ **Sotol Overlook**

Wildcat Canyon Trail

Far Reaches Trail

Senderos Balcones Trail

L A U R E L   C A N Y O N

Joe Johnston Route

Chula Vista

Bluff Spurs Trail

Laurel Canyon Trail

Recharge Trail

visitor center ■

Klepper Way

savanna restoration area

FEET						
1,400						
1,350						
1,300						
1,250						
1,200						
1,150						
1,100						
1,050						
1,000	1	2	3	4	5	6	7

MILES

Chula Vista

Antonio. The views keep coming on your descent. Your return trip straddles the margin between the Balcones Escarpment and the flatter savanna restoration area. Be apprised that the trail is open to both hikers and mountain bikers.

Leave the visitor center, joining a gravel trail leading east to meet Klepper Way and a road bridge over Government Canyon. Beyond the road bridge, immediately reach the backcountry trailhead and then turn left, picking up the historic Joe Johnston Route. The modern trail is overlaid on a military road from the 1850s. After a quarter mile you will meet the Recharge Trail and the loop portion of your hike. Stay forward, still on the Joe Johnston Route, bordered by juniper on a rocky doubletrack, mostly open to the sun. Cross Government Canyon wash and then pass a spur trail leading left to the Wildcat Canyon Ranch structures. Bobcats, coyotes, and javelinas now patrol this former cattle country.

Reach a clearing and the Wildcat Canyon Trail at 1.1 miles. Immediately step over Government Canyon wash to enter Wildcat Canyon. Live oaks, junipers, and scattered grasses border the trail. Hills flank the track. Saddle alongside the Wildcat Canyon wash at 1.5 miles. Note how the trees near the wash point downstream, reflecting the sporadic torrents that pour through this valley. Gently ascend, occasionally crossing braids of the wash in tree thickets. At 2.3 miles, leave the canyon bottom and climb away on a rocky track. The less moist environment is reflected in the correspondent shrubby nature of the trees. Reach the High Lonesome Windmill at 2.6 miles. The blades are gone from the windmill, and the structure is now used

Winter offers far-reaching views.

as a park antenna tower. Continue wandering through a hodgepodge of grass and rock glens interspersed with evergreen patches.

Intersect the Sendero Balcones Trail at 2.8 miles. Tired hikers can shortcut the loop by heading south here. However, the main hike keeps forward, joining the Far Reaches Trail and circling the head of Laurel Canyon. The rocky tread resembles pieces of a jigsaw puzzle. Meet the spur trail leading left to Sotol Overlook at 3.2 miles. The vista point offers views of the immediate natural area, with distant hills and civilization to the south and east. More views open ahead. A clear winter day will afford looks to the east, south, and west. Keep working mostly downhill to reach Chula Vista at 4.4 miles. The easterly views are unparalleled. You have a commanding view of San Antonio. This visit is worth having a seat at the strategically located bench. A stony downgrade reaches the flatlands at 5.2 miles. Turn right here, westbound, traveling the fault line where water enters the Edwards Aquifer. Bisect a dry wash at 5.3 miles, and pass the closed Laurel Canyon Trail at 5.6 miles. Curve south and then meet the Recharge Trail at 5.7 miles. Pick up a westbound doubletrack. Enjoy traveling the nexus of hill and prairie, with the savanna restoration to your left.

The grasslands that once stretched across central Texas were what attracted settlers in the first place, with wavy meadows and prairies providing nourishment for livestock. Sam Houston reported about Texas to Andrew Jackson, "I have no hesitancy in pronouncing it the finest country to its extent on the globe . . . there can be no doubt but the country east of the Rio Grande would sustain a population of ten million souls." Texas has more than doubled that. However, with the settling of the land came overgrazing, fencing, and fire suppression, which in the end altered the ecosystem from grassland to cedar and in other cases dirt and rock. That is why the savanna restoration is important, to return the land to a semblance of what it looked like when the precursors of today's visitors first laid eyes on Government Canyon and the lands around it.

Intersect the Sendero Balcones Trail at 6.3 miles. Keep west on the Recharge Trail, passing the campground access trail and then the Bluff Spurs Trail, reaching Joe Johnston Route at 6.9 miles, completing the loop. Backtrack to the trailhead.

NEARBY ACTIVITIES

Government Canyon State Natural Area offers drive-up tent and RV camping, backcountry camping, and picnic facilities.

COMANCHE LOOKOUT LOOP 42

IN BRIEF

This hike travels up to and around a historic hill northeast of San Antonio in a suburban park. The trail surface varies from asphalt to gravel to concrete as it ascends to an old tower with stupendous views of San Antonio and then circles around the hill.

DESCRIPTION

What once was an eclectic residence on the edge of town, and before that a Native American watch post, has now turned into a suburban park, where residents can enjoy a vista purely for pleasure and get a little exercise in the meantime. The hike leaves the trailhead on busy Nacogdoches Road and follows a paved path up to Comanche Lookout, where you can see the surprisingly tall tower of the former residence. From here, circle down and around a hill to make a surprisingly rewarding and invigorating hike. If the distance is a bit short for your taste, just do the hike all over again, or make your own trek using the myriad gravel paths that wind throughout the park.

The unnamed paved path leaves the trailhead and begins a rise through scattered juniper and mesquite trees. A concrete path soon leaves to the left. This is your return route. Keep following the asphalt trail uphill, passing a second concrete path crossing the asphalt trail. Before too long the asphalt path makes a

KEY AT-A-GLANCE INFORMATION

LENGTH: 1.7 miles

CONFIGURATION: Loop

DIFFICULTY: Moderate

SCENERY: Cedar forest, hilltop vistas

EXPOSURE: Mostly open

TRAFFIC: Moderate–busy on weekends

TRAIL SURFACE: Asphalt, gravel, concrete

HIKING TIME: 1.3 hours

DRIVING DISTANCE: 17 miles from the Alamo

ACCESS: Daily, 5 a.m.–11 p.m.; no fees or permits

WHEELCHAIR ACCESS: Yes, on paved part of hike

MAPS: sanantonio.gov/sapar/pdf/ Comanche_Lookout_trails.pdf

FACILITIES: Water fountain near old tower

CONTACT INFORMATION: (210) 207-8480; sanantonio.gov/sapar

Directions

From Exit 172 on I-35 north of San Antonio, take Loop 1604 west 1.5 miles to FR 2252, Nacogdoches Road. Head west on Nacogdoches toward San Antonio, 1 mile. The trailhead at Comanche Lookout Park will be on your right.

GPS TRAILHEAD COORDINATES

LATITUDE: 29° 58' 29.17"
LONGITUDE: 98° 36' 64.72"

COMANCHE
LOOKOUT PARK

Fox Run
Elementary School

Rocky Creek Road

Fox Creek Street

Timberway Street

Oak Country Way

Nacogdoches Road

Falcon Crest

Vigil View

To
Loop 1604

FM 2252

N

0   250   500
feet

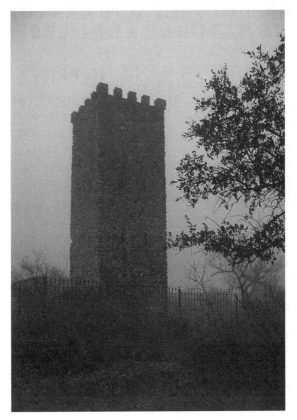
Stone tower atop Comanche Lookout

turnaround atop the hill. From here, head south and the old tower comes into view.

Comanche Lookout is the fourth-highest point in Bexar County at 1,340 feet. The Apache, then the Comanche, used the hill as a vantage point for warfare and hunting. It was also a landmark for travelers in the 1700s. The Camino Real, which led from San Antonio to Nacogdoches, traveled past the hill. Your access road, Nacogdoches Road, traces the old Camino Real.

Comanche Lookout changed hands several times after Texas was settled. In 1923 Edward H. Coppack, a history buff, bought the land and envisioned a medieval-style castle atop the hill. His compound included a four-story stone tower. After Coppack died his children sold the land to a developer, who tore down all but the stone tower, which still stands today. In the early 1990s, a movement to save Comanche Lookout was born, resulting in the city of San Antonio acquiring the 92 acres and developing it as a park (with plans for more).

The old tower is now fenced in. However, for a good view, keep along the ridgeline heading south, past the lookout. In places, live oak trees thrive, but a clearing at the south tip of the hilltop affords an excellent and far-reaching vista of the greater San Antonio area. Curve around from the south point, passing the lookout a second time. Here, a side trail curves downhill, crossing the asphalt trail you took to the top. Keep on a downgrade, passing Fox Run Elementary School to your right. Reach a low point at Fox Run Road. A normally dry creek bed lies to your right.

Keep curving around the hill. The forest gives way, and you can look toward the hilltop. A short loop has been added, which connects to an outdoor classroom. All too soon the path intersects the asphalt trail near the trailhead. Walk a few steps back to the parking area and complete the loop.

43   CROWNRIDGE CANYON NATURAL AREA LOOP

KEY AT-A-GLANCE INFORMATION

LENGTH: 1.9 miles

CONFIGURATION: Loop

DIFFICULTY: Easy to moderate

SCENERY: Open and wooded hills

EXPOSURE: Partly open

TRAFFIC: Busy on nice days

TRAIL SURFACE: Compressed gravel, natural surfaces

HIKING TIME: 1.3 hours

DRIVING DISTANCE: 19 miles from the Alamo

ACCESS: No fee required; no pets allowed

WHEELCHAIR ACCESS: Yes, on lower loop

MAPS: sanaturalareas.org/cr/ crtrails.html

FACILITIES: Restrooms, water, picnicking at trailhead

CONTACT INFORMATION: (210) 207-8480; sanaturalareas.org/cr/ crindex.html

GPS TRAILHEAD COORDINATES

LATITUDE: 29° 36' 58.83"
LONGITUDE: 98° 37' 50.14"

IN BRIEF

This recently developed city of San Antonio designated natural area offers an excellent loop hike in a canyon that serves as a recharge zone for the Edwards Aquifer and a repository for native flora and fauna.

DESCRIPTION

The city of San Antonio has recognized the need to protect its water supply for an expanding population. At the same time, it also realized that recreation areas can benefit the population as a whole, providing exercise outlets in a visually appealing area while preserving natural beauty, which has its own intangible benefits. Crownridge Canyon Natural Area addresses all of the above. The preserve is part of an effort to replenish the Edwards Aquifer, which provides water for greater San Antonio, the largest city in the country to use an underground aquifer for its main water source. Protecting and recharging this aquifer is vital to the citizens who live here. This natural area is but 200 acres, yet it helps by allowing water to percolate into the soil, rather than taking it out if it were developed. Furthermore, the natural area shelters disappearing habitat and provides a place to

---

Directions ⸻⟶

From the intersection of Loop 1604 and I-10 northwest of downtown San Antonio, take I-10 west toward El Paso to Exit 554, Camp Bullis Road. Turn left on Camp Bullis Road, passing under the interstate, heading west. At 1.6 miles turn right on Luskey Road. It is a quick right onto a downhill before a bridge, so be ready. Follow Luskey Road for 0.3 miles, then turn right into Crownridge Canyon Natural Area.

Bear Grass Trail

Red Oak
Canyon Bridge

Bear Grass
Falls

Wagner Way

Red Oak Trail

Luskey Boulevard

To
10 87

Babcock Road

Camp Bluffs Road

Crownridge Canyon displays restored
Hill Country habitat.

restore habitat that once was here. Simply put, the closer you are to downtown
San Antonio the more likely a given area is going to be developed. Crownridge
Canyon gives flora and fauna a place to thrive. But it wasn't always this way—
for years the canyon was used as a dump. After the land was purchased by the
city, the trash was removed and then an ongoing effort began to restore the
habitat to its condition prior to the arrival of European settlers. The Texas Hill
Country was once vast grassland, scattered with trees. However, fire was sup-
pressed as settlements grew, allowing the oaks and junipers to take over, which
is much of what we see today. However, fire, tree removal, and native plant
restoration are being used in concert at Crownridge Canyon to replicate what
this land once was, giving Crownridge Canyon a dual benefit.

For hikers there is yet another benefit—a trail system comprised of two
interconnected loops. Red Oak Trail is the lower loop. The hard-packed surface
allows wheelchair access for its entire length. Bear Grass Trail is a natural surface
upper loop that offers foot travelers a deeper look into the canyon. During wetter
times, when the canyon stream flows, trailed treaders will enjoy Bear Grass Falls,
a cascade that drops over a stone lip into a rocky pool.

Your experience begins at the trailhead, where a shaded interpretive area
explains the importance of places such as Crownridge Canyon. The information
illuminates the human and natural history of the area and the importance of the
Edwards Aquifer. Walk just a short distance and come to the loop portion of the

hike. Take a left, switchbacking up the canyon's west side. Cedars and oaks shade much of the trail, but this park is grassier than most because of the ongoing savanna restoration. Contemplation benches are situated throughout the trail system. Soon views of the Texas Hill Country open up, with houses at the uppermost reaches of the canyon. Continue up the trail, reaching Red Oak Canyon Bridge at 0.5 mile. If water is running in the creek bed, you stand a good chance of seeing Bear Grass Falls in action.

At 0.7 mile you'll reach Bear Grass Trail. It continues forward as a narrower natural-surface trail, while Red Oak Trail leads right to make a 1.3-mile loop. Enter the upper canyon, dipping into a drainage, then ascend under a tight tree canopy on a stony path. Enjoy the rugged trek as it cuts down the canyon amid deciduous oaks. Circle just above Bear Grass Falls at 1.4 miles. If it is running, you will have to rock-hop the stream. The trail widens and intersects Red Oak Trail beyond Bear Grass Falls. Meander with the canyon bottom to your left and scattered grasslands to your right. Savanna restoration is abundant here, as well as the re-plantation of native elm, walnut, cherry, and native grasses. Restoring the ecosystem to its natural state also strengthens the habitat for native fauna, which evolved to depend on the plants and their fruits for food. At 1.6 miles cross Red Oak Canyon and continue drifting through a mosaic of grass and trees before completing the hike at 1.9 miles.

44 FRIEDRICH PARK TRAIL

KEY AT-A-GLANCE INFORMATION

LENGTH: 2.3 miles

CONFIGURATION: Loop

DIFFICULTY: Difficult

SCENERY: Thick hardwoods, limestone, endangered songbirds

EXPOSURE: Shady

TRAFFIC: Light

TRAIL SURFACE: Concrete, dirt, roots, rock

HIKING TIME: 1.5 hours

DRIVING DISTANCE: 19 miles from the Alamo

ACCESS: Daily, 7:30 a.m.–sunset; closed Christmas and New Year's Day; no fees or permits

WHEELCHAIR ACCESS: Yes, in some areas

MAPS: sanaturalareas.org/fp/fptrails.html

FACILITIES: Restrooms

CONTACT INFORMATION: (210) 207-8480; sanaturalareas.org/fp/fpindex.html

GPS TRAILHEAD COORDINATES

LATITUDE: 29° 63' 96.94"
LONGITUDE: 98° 62' 63.33"

IN BRIEF

This is a rugged hike in a pristine Hill Country preserve with a 350-foot climb, steep and narrow trails, and an abundance of Texas plant life. The Friedrich Wilderness Park is also home to one of the oldest working windmills in Bexar County.

DESCRIPTION

If not for Norma Friedrich Ward, the 232-acre Friedrich Wilderness Park would not be a reality. In 1971 Ward bequeathed 180 acres of this land to the city of San Antonio in memory of her parents to ensure that the native vegetation and wildlife would be protected. W.L. Mathews and Associates donated an additional 52 adjacent acres. Now the Friends of Friedrich Wilderness Park, in conjunction with San Antonio Parks and Recreation, maintains a stewardship role to this unique resource that offers more than 5 miles of trails.

Unlike some local parks, Friedrich Wilderness Park has an extensive trail system open to wheelchairs. Each trail is rated, indicating how appropriate it is for wheelchair use. Levels 1 through 3 are open to wheelchairs and indicate increasing difficulty. Level 1 trails have gentle slopes and are paved with either asphalt or concrete, whereas Level 3 trails consist of crushed-stone surface and slopes are significantly steeper. Wheelchair users are cautioned that exceptional upper-body strength

- -

Directions ⟶

Take I-10 West from San Antonio, and then take Exit 554 to Camp Bullis Road. Stay on the access road until you can turn west on Oak. When you reach the end of Oak, turn north—the park is on the left.

may be required. Level 4 trails are unimproved dirt designed to be difficult to traverse. They may include rock ledges and steep gradients and are not accessible to wheelchairs.

The trailhead at the southwest end of the parking lot provides access to all of the park's trails. You'll see a bulletin board and kiosk with information about the park, as well as a desk with a Plexiglas cover containing trail maps, a bird list, and a guest book for visitors to sign.

A flyer titled "Emilie and Albert Friedrich Wilderness Park" also contains a trail map and interpretive information to correspond with numbered points along the various trails. This is easier to read and carry than the photocopied map.

Start your hike by heading west on the concrete Main Loop Trail. The shade provided by the trees helps make this hike a little more bearable on an otherwise hot day. Numerous benches are located at the beginning legs of the trail. You'll reach a T-intersection about 450 feet into the trail. The Forest Range Trail takes off to the right, and the Main Loop, designated as a Level 2 trail from this point on, continues to the left.

The trail changes from concrete to asphalt as it continues up the hill and across a wooden bridge over a dry creek bed. Several sections of fencing are visible on your right, but it is unclear what purpose they serve. Another T-intersection is reached at 0.3 miles. You will return to this point later using the trail on your right, so head left to continue on the southern portion of the Main Loop Trail. The trail surface turns to mulch as you keep traveling the Main Loop, and the incline starts to increase. The trail forks 300 feet ahead. Continue on the Main Loop Trail, or go right on the more rugged, Level 4 Water Trail, which rejoins the Main Loop. About 0.1 mile past the intersection of the Main Loop and Water Trail, you'll reach the Juniper Barrens Loop Trail, which appears on your left. Continue right along the Main Loop Trail, which becomes a Level 4 trail from this point. The trail surface is dirt and rock from here on.

As the incline steadily increases, you'll see a bench on the left; this is the last place to sit for a while. After you've climbed about 200 feet (to 1,390 feet elevation), a sign informs hikers that the remainder of the park has been set aside as protected habitat for the black-capped vireo. These small songbirds make nests from the bark strips of the ash juniper tree (also called the mountain cedar) found in this area. One of the main reasons for the vireo's decline is habitat loss, though they also fall prey to the parasitic nesting of the brown-headed cowbird. These larger birds lay their eggs in other birds' nests and abandon them to be raised by the nest's owners. The young cowbirds usually hatch first and crowd out the other chicks.

You'll come to another sign with the park's map system on it and find a fork in the trail. The Main Loop continues to the right, but go left on Vista Loop Trail, which rejoins the Main Loop in about a mile. Go up the hill to reach the park's highest point (1,440 feet) 1 mile into the hike. Enjoy the great views of the surrounding area. Nearby you will see a wall constructed of stacked limestone that crosses the trail and disappears north into the brush. The trail leaves the wall behind, becomes very narrow and rocky, and soon loops back to rejoin the wall, turning north to follow the rock wall for several tenths of a mile. Shortly after rejoining the wall, you'll come to an intersection with the Upland Range Trail, which leads 0.1 mile back to the Main Loop Trail. Stay on the Vista Loop Trail.

The trail is now on the backside of the hill you just climbed, and the view to the west is expansive. Miles of hills and valleys roll on with very little sign of civilization. You'll reach another sign about the black-capped vireo habitat and shortly thereafter see a set of earthen stairs leading down. The dirt and root surface of the trail requires that you watch your step. The trail is very narrow at this point, and steep gradients leave no room for error on the left side. Occasionally wooden planks have been added to shore up the trail against erosion. Another set of earth-and-wood stairs at just over 1.5 miles leads down into and back out of a small canyon.

Shortly after the stairs, you'll reach the Fern Del Trail on your right. If you haven't felt challenged enough, take this short, steep loop trail, which rejoins Vista Loop Trail. Otherwise continue on, passing the other end of Fern Del Trail 0.1 mile later. You'll soon meet back up with the Main Loop trail and a sign noting that you are 0.5 miles from the trailhead. Turn left and go mostly downhill from this point. Having climbed back out of the valley in which you were, you'll be able to hear the traffic that was inaudible on the opposite side of the hill.

The hike ends on the same trail on which it began, and the downhill slope is a welcome change. The cement trail leads back to the parking lot, past the kiosk you passed on the way into the park. Sign the guest book if you haven't already, and be sure to note any birds you may have sighted in their log.

The Friedrich Wilderness Park is a very delicate ecosystem, and rules require that it be treated as such. No pets or bicycles are allowed, and fires and smoking are also prohibited.

45 GOVERNMENT CANYON LOOP

KEY AT-A-GLANCE INFORMATION

LENGTH: 6.4 miles

CONFIGURATION: Balloon loop

DIFFICULTY: Moderate–difficult

SCENERY: Open and wooded canyon

EXPOSURE: Partly open

TRAFFIC: Busy on nice days

TRAIL SURFACE: Natural surfaces

HIKING TIME: 3.5 hours

DRIVING DISTANCE: 25 miles from the Alamo

ACCESS: Friday–Monday, 7 a.m.–10 p.m.; $6/person over age 13

WHEELCHAIR ACCESS: No

MAPS: tpwd.state.tx.us/publications

CONTACT INFORMATION: (210) 688-9055; tpwd.state.tx.us/spdest/findadest/parks/government_canyon

GPS TRAILHEAD COORDINATES

LATITUDE: 29° 32' 55.00"
LONGITUDE: 98° 45' 54.20"

IN BRIEF

This hike bisects the heart of Government Canyon, a state natural area. Travel past historic ranch buildings to reach a canyon overlook before looping to a stone house above watery springs. Finally, wander into a live oak and Spanish moss garden that aboriginal Texans called home.

DESCRIPTION

Government Canyon State Natural Area was set aside for protecting and recharging the Edwards Aquifer, which provides San Antonio its drinking water. The 8,000-plus-acre preserve also provides a large swath of public land for hikers to explore. Opened in 2005, the park facilities continue to expand, with the inclusion of frontcountry and backcountry camping and the restoration of natural ecosystems. *Note:* Most of this circuit is open to both mountain bikers and hikers.

This particular track enters the heart of Government Canyon, crisscrossing the rocky wash bordered by dense woods, grassy areas, and rock bluffs. Visit the old Wildcat Canyon Ranch structures before pushing deeper into the canyon and reaching the loop portion of the hike. Here you will join a singletrack path as it climbs the canyon walls, making an overlook

----

Directions

From the intersection of Loop 1604 and Shaenfield Road, northwest of downtown and south of Braun Road, take Shaenfield Road west for 1.6 miles to a traffic light. Continue forward through the light as Shaenfield Road becomes Galm Road. Keep west on Galm Road and follow it 1.9 miles to the entrance on your right. Once in the park, drive to the visitor center. The trails begin there.

45 Government Canyon Loop

N

0   0.25   0.5
mile

Overlook Trail

Caroline's Loop

Little Windmill Trail

Senderos Balcones Trail

Zizelmann House

Canyon Overlook

Twin Oaks Trail

Wildcat Canyon Trail

Hoffman Hayfield

Joe Johnston Route

Senderos Balcones Trail

Laurel Canyon Trail

Wildcat Canyon Ranch Buildings

Bluff Spurs Trail

Recharge Trail

savanna restoration area

visitor center

Klepper Way

P

Clear pools lie below this canyon overlook.

atop a sheer rock bluff. Views extend up and down the canyon and into Texas Hill Country beyond. The circuit then drops to reach the Zizelmann House, a stone Texas-style dwelling situated near Government Canyon Springs. On your return trip, you'll visit the village site of the first Texans, who lived in Government Canyon under a scenic live oak copse with a concentration of Spanish moss, giving it a magical look. Saunter underneath more canyon walls before backtracking to the trailhead.

Leave the parking area and make your way to the visitor center. Interesting interpretive information and helpful staff are on hand to enhance your hiking adventure. Head right, passing a display about the Edwards Aquifer, and then join a gravel path heading east to briefly join Klepper Way, crossing Government Canyon on a road bridge. Immediately reach the backcountry trailhead. Turn left here and trace the Joe Johnston Route, an old northbound doubletrack heading up Government Canyon. It was originally cut as a military road connecting San Antonio to Bandera in the 1850s, and it later became a ranch road.

Meet the Recharge Trail a quarter mile from the trailhead. All trails and intersections are clearly marked. Keep forward on an often-rocky Joe Johnston Route. At 0.5 miles traverse the canyon wash, entering a forest of cedar, elm, scrub oaks, and mountain laurel. Intermittent streambeds cut into the main canyon across the historic road. At 0.9 miles a short spur trail leads left to the Wildcat Canyon Ranch buildings. Vegetation is growing up around the wood-and-metal structures. Continue up the Joe Johnston Route to reach a clearing and a trail junction at 1.1 miles. Here the Wildcat Canyon Trail leads right. This hike keeps forward on a canopied track between crisscrossing washes. Look for steep canyon walls to your left. The old Hoffman Hayfield lies below distant cliffs at 1.9 miles.

Spanish moss gives the trail a magical look.

Gently rise through live oaks to reach the Twin Oaks Trail at 2.2 miles. Keep forward, soon crossing Government Canyon wash yet again, and meet a junction at 2.5 miles. Here Caroline's Loop and the Overlook Trail leave left while the Joe Johnston Route keeps forward. Stay left with Caroline's Loop–Overlook Trail and then split right with the hiker-only Overlook Trail at 2.6 miles. Climb through scrubby cedars and cacti, crossing small washes to reach an open cliff top and the Canyon Overlook at 2.9 miles. Look down on Government Canyon, which should have water here and at the hilly wildlands beyond. More overlooks ahead allow for multiple vistas. The Overlook Trail falls into Government Canyon after crossing a few dry washes to reach a flat and a trail junction near the Zizelmann House at 3.5 miles. It is unclear if anyone ever lived in this house, but the classic central Texas stone ranch structure will hopefully be stabilized and able to explore in the future. But for now it's encircled by fence. However, you can walk around the area, as well as see an old well and take a trail down to the canyon wash, where springs are likely to be flowing.

From the Zizelmann House, turn right, heading southwesterly, back on the Joe Johnston Route. It isn't long before you enter the live oak and Spanish moss garden, where an irregular surface indicates past archaeological digging. The alluring locale was home to aboriginal Texans. Cross Government Canyon just below the Canyon Overlook. Relish a bottom-up view of the overhanging cliff on which you were standing earlier. Complete the loop portion of the hike at 3.9 miles and then backtrack 2.5 miles down the Joe Johnston Route to the trailhead.

NEARBY ACTIVITIES

Government Canyon State Natural Area offers drive-up tent and RV camping, backcountry camping, and picnic facilities.

46 HILL VIEW TRAIL

KEY AT-A-GLANCE INFORMATION

LENGTH: 3.2 miles

CONFIGURATION: Loop with balloon spur

DIFFICULTY: Moderate

SCENERY: Typical Hill Country woodland, abundant wildlife, dog lovers

EXPOSURE: Mostly shady

TRAFFIC: Moderate

TRAIL SURFACE: Cement, rock, asphalt, dirt

HIKING TIME: 1.5 hours

DRIVING DISTANCE: 19 miles from the Alamo

ACCESS: Daily, 6 a.m.–sunset; closed Christmas and New Year's Day; no fees or permits

WHEELCHAIR ACCESS: Yes, but only at trail's beginning

MAPS: sanaturalareas.org/ep/eptrails.html

FACILITIES: Picnic tables, restrooms

CONTACT INFORMATION: (210) 207-8480; sanaturalareas.org/ep/epindex.html

GPS TRAILHEAD COORDINATES

LATITUDE: 29° 62' 50.56"
LONGITUDE: 98° 57' 09.44"

IN BRIEF

Located north of San Antonio, this wild area serves as a retreat for bikers, joggers, and hikers. Pet lovers can also enjoy this hike through natural Hill Country woodland that includes a stop at an observation tower overlooking the city.

DESCRIPTION

Dwight D. Eisenhower Park is just one more of the many wild places located within a stone's throw of the city. In fact, it is a designated city natural area, increasing in popularity. Even weekday evenings bring out a good number of people looking to get away from the bustle of the workday.

Note: Camp Bullis Training Site, a military reservation, borders the park, so don't cross any fences. Bicyclers use the park, so watch for them as you enter.

The hike begins in the large group picnic area on the south side of the park. Wherever you wind up parking, you'll be walking south to get to the trailhead. A birthday party or company picnic is usually going on here, so looking for the crowd can be just as effective. A restroom is located between the lot and the pavilion that serves as party headquarters. Don't let the crowds dissuade you; things will get much quieter soon.

Follow the signs to the Hill View Trail, and walk behind and to the right of the picnic area. The trail at this point is cement and part

----

Directions

From Exit 558 on I-10 north of San Antonio, take Loop Road 1604 eastbound to Northwest Military Highway. Exit from Loop Road 160 north on Northwest Military Highway and follow it 2 miles north to the trailhead.

N

0   0.1   0.2
mile

N.W. Military Hwy.

radio tower

substations

P

Hill View Trail

Shady Creek Trail

Cedar Flats Trail

EISENHOWER PARK

Yucca Flats Trail

bat houses

Live Oak Trail

Hill View Trail

tower

FEET

1,400
1,350
1,300
1,250
1,200
1,150
1,100
1,050
1,000

0.5   1   1.5   2   2.5   3   3.2

MILES

of a larger trail system. The trail forks 0.2 miles into the hike, where directional signs show the choices before you. To the left lies a rock trail named Hill View N (for natural). The other trail is the Hill View paved trail that continues forward to an exit in the parking lot and back from where you came. Take the trail to the left to get off the beaten path.

The surrounding hillside is typical of the terrain first encountered by settlers arriving in this area of Texas, and it looks deceptively fertile. However, the dense mesquite, hackberry, and cedar—as well as the thriving saw grass and yucca—hide the rocky soil, which is of little use for farming. The inhospitable soil is what steered the early settlers toward the sheep and cattle industries. With the exception of grazing, there's not much more this land will support.

Keep hiking down the trail until you see a spur that looks more like a game trail than a hiking trail. Ignore this path, which leads to the off-limits military reservation, and continue a little farther until you reach a junction just over 0.5 miles into the hike. This one is legitimate and is clearly marked. The Shady Creek Trail to the left is a short loop off the paved Cedar Flats Trail that will reconnect with this trail farther ahead. Stay on the path you're on for now. Soon the second Shady Creek junction joins the trail. At this point turn to the left and take the Shady Creek Trail.

This trail joins the paved Cedar Flats Trail in about 350 yards. Take the Cedar Flats Trail to the right, and start toward the observation tower at the top of the hill.

Located at an intersection of three trails, the observation area sits 1.2 miles into your trek. Here the natural Yucca Flats Trail (to the right) leads to permit-only campsites and eventually loops back into the parking area to the left. The Live Oak Trail, also a natural surface, leads straight ahead and up the hill, joining the Hill View loop south of the observation tower. The third trail is the Cedar Flats Trail, and it, too, continues up the hill and takes you to the tower.

On the left side of the trail, partially obscured by a large tree, sit two benches overlooking a clearing on the opposite side of the trail. Look for the white plywood banners marked with a bat silhouette—nearby shelters help attract bats to the area, but their presence is not as reliable as in other areas of the state.

Just past the benches, the Cedar Flats Trail intersects the Hill View Trail, on which the hike began, at 1.3 miles. Signs mark the trails at the junctions, and a restroom stands on the left side of the paved trail. From this point the Cedar Flats Trail continues toward a small loop and the observation tower. The Hill View Trail loops back toward the trailhead at both ends. Continue up the paved trail for 0.1 mile to visit the tower. The Holly Hills Optimist Club built this wooden structure in 1984, and it shows minimal wear after so many years. Constructed of 4- x 4-inch beams, it resembles the modern play areas found in most parks these days, and a staircase leads up two flights to the observation platform. The view from here is vast, to say the least. At 1,290 feet, this is the high point of the park. The view encompasses the rolling hills to the north and west, as well as San Antonio to the south. Loop 1604 and its traffic are visible 2 miles south of the park. A large quarry operation is also visible from the tower.

After taking a break to enjoy the view, return down the Cedar Flats Trail to the junction with the Hill View Trail. From this point, remaining on the paved trail will take you back downhill to the trailheads and parking lot. The Hill View loop to the right takes a roundabout path to the same destination and offers a chance to view more of the bird and animal life of the park. Follow the natural Hill View Trail to the right.

Depending on the time of day, the chances of seeing white-tailed deer coming out of their hiding places are very good. On most hikes here, I've been able to hike within a few yards of the wary creatures. Cottontail rabbits, roadrunners, and even wild hogs can also be seen among the yucca, mesquite, and prickly pear.

The trail surface switches from rock to dirt and is very easy to traverse at this point in the hike, which meanders downhill for the rest. Joggers and dog walkers just beginning their hikes start to appear from down the trail. At 1.7 miles into the hike, a spur to the left, marked by a sign as the Live Oak Trail, leads into the thick and eventually joins the Cedar Flats Trail.

At 2.2 miles the trail meets with a high fence, which it parallels for the remainder of the hike, and turns left. This begins the last leg of the hike, and the trail is mostly level from this point on. High-current power lines buzz overhead, carrying their load to a transformer station across the street from the park. Three miles into the hike you'll see the park's baseball field on the other side of the fence. A concrete jogging trail is also visible to the left. The trail ends in the pavilion area in which it began, just a few yards from the map sign.

47 LEON CREEK VISTA AT O.P. SCHNABEL PARK

KEY AT-A-GLANCE INFORMATION

LENGTH: 1.2 miles

CONFIGURATION: Loop

DIFFICULTY: Easy

SCENERY: Cedar forest, bluff

EXPOSURE: Mostly shady

TRAFFIC: Very heavy

TRAIL SURFACE: Concrete

HIKING TIME: 1 hour

DRIVING DISTANCE: 16 miles from the Alamo

ACCESS: Daily, 5 a.m.–11 p.m.; no fees or permits

WHEELCHAIR ACCESS: Yes

MAPS: sanantonio.gov/sapar/pdf/ opschnabeltrails.pdf

FACILITIES: Restrooms, water, play area, pavilion at trailhead

CONTACT INFORMATION: (210) 207-8480; sanantonio.gov/sapar

GPS TRAILHEAD COORDINATES

LATITUDE: 29° 53' 37.22"
LONGITUDE: 98° 64' 15.56"

IN BRIEF

This walk makes a loop at one of San Antonio's most visited parks. Often used by walkers, bikers, and dog enthusiasts, this trail curves along the bluffs overlooking Leon Creek, where you can view the city. An additional concrete walkway winds through other parts of the park.

DESCRIPTION

This walking trail is convenient for those living in San Antonio northwest of downtown. O.P. Schnabel Park is well maintained and attractive, offering many other activities in addition to walking. The trail makes a convenient loop amid fine scenery and is topped off with a good view. The convenience and attractiveness draw the crowds, though. On weekend afternoons you may be hard-pressed to find a parking spot. Despite the crowds, the trail has its regulars who walk, jog, or lead their dogs. Try to hit this spot on the off-times and it may become part of your routine. Be aware that mountain bikers will be plying the myriad dirt trails spurring off the paved and concrete loop.

In 1964 the city of San Antonio purchased this property where French Creek runs south, eventually meeting Leon Creek downstream. The many oaks were the initial drawing card at

Directions

From the junction of Loop 1604, Anderson Loop, and TX 16 Bandera Road, head south on Bandera Road for 1.7 miles to the O. P. Schnabel Park entrance on your left. Turn into the park and reach a T-intersection. Turn left and you'll shortly reach the Sadie Ray and Waldo Graff Pavilion. The trail starts near the pavilion.

what was then called Bandera Road Park. In 1977 the park was renamed after O.P. Schnabel. He had built a reputation in town for his anti-litter campaigns based on such sayings as "nice people don't litter," and "be a beauty bug, not a litterbug." His detractors said his initials stood for "Old Pushbroom." Schnabel's good works live on at the Beautify San Antonio Association, which he helped found. Today, housing developments have sprung up both north and south of the park, leaving the park as a nice little suburban niche of green amid the sprawl. Ball fields, picnic areas, and additional paved trails have been built, attracting even more visitors.

Leave the Sadie Ray and Waldo Graff Pavilion on an asphalt trail. Immediately turn left onto a concrete path. Keep alongside a picnic and play area. A mixture of cedar, oak, and grass lines the path. At 0.2 miles, the trail runs into a T-intersection at the park's northern edge. Houses back up to the park fence. Turn right here, climbing slightly. Come around to reach a high point near a transmission tower. Pass alongside the tower. Gain views from the bluffs that you are straddling. At 0.5 miles reach a tin-roofed pavilion. A concrete side trail leads to a cleared overlook. The valley of Leon Creek lies below, and the bulk of San Antonio spreads out to the south and east.

Keep south on the bluff line beyond the overlook. Many dirt spurs dip off the bluff. Curve away from the bluff line as you approach the houses on Tippit Trail. The path begins to curve back toward the parking area. Meander west and then north beneath cedar trees thick enough to provide more-than-adequate shade. Pass a path that shortcuts the main loop. Return to the parking area and complete the loop. You are at the south end of the large parking area near the pavilion.

If you are interested in doing a little more walking, look for the concrete trail leading away from the pavilion back toward Bandera Road. The trail immediately crosses the park road near the pavilion and heads around park facilities to loop across French Creek.

McALLISTER PARK TRAIL 48

IN BRIEF

A lot of things go into making a good hike, and McAllister Park has most of them. Location, accessibility, flora, and fauna combine to make this trail, located right in San Antonio, well worth the trip.

DESCRIPTION

Located on the north side of town near San Antonio International Airport, this 856-acre park is well maintained. Apparently, few people know about its existence, but those who do use it often. Although no official trailhead exists, the path can be accessed from numerous parking areas, allowing you to shorten your hike if you don't have time to walk the whole length.

To get the most distance out of the trail system here, this hike starts at the southeast corner of the park. Only a few places allow you to double back on previously hiked sections. After parking, walk toward the baseball fields until you see the trailhead on your left. This is where you'll start.

The trees grow close to the trail, and there is little room off either side of the path to wander unimpeded. Wide enough to walk two abreast or to allow joggers and bicyclists to pass the slower walkers, the paved trail is well shaded and allows a feeling of solitude for most of the hike.

As you make your way along the trail, you'll reach a T-intersection. The trail to the right leads around the baseball fields and

KEY AT-A-GLANCE INFORMATION

LENGTH: 3.6 miles

CONFIGURATION: Figure eight

DIFFICULTY: Easy

SCENERY: Thick woodland park with an abundance of wildlife

EXPOSURE: Shady

TRAFFIC: Heavy

TRAIL SURFACE: Asphalt

HIKING TIME: 1.7 hours

DRIVING DISTANCE: 12 miles from the Alamo

ACCESS: Daily, 5 a.m.–11 p.m.; no fees or permits

WHEELCHAIR ACCESS: Yes

MAPS: sanantonio.gov/sapar/pdf/ mcallistermaprevised.pdf

FACILITIES: Restrooms and water fountains at the main pavilion

CONTACT INFORMATION: (210) 207-8480; sanantonio.gov/sapar

Directions

From US 281 in San Antonio, turn east on Nakoma Street, which becomes Jones Maltsberger Road. Continue about 1.5 miles, and the park will be on your right.

GPS TRAILHEAD COORDINATES

LATITUDE: 29° 55' 00.00"
LONGITUDE: 98° 44' 42.78"

N

0   0.2   0.4
mile

Jones Maltsberger Road

Thousand Oaks Drive

Mud Creek

Turkey Roost

Buckhorn

Soccer

police station

Leaping Fawn

Lorence Creek

P

Buckhorn

McALLISTER PARK

Starcrest Drive

FEET

900
850
800
750
700
650
600
550
500

0.5   1   1.5   2   2.5   3   3.6

MILES

rejoins one of the loops. Take the trail to the left. At 0.7 miles into the trek, you'll see the pavilions you passed when you drove into the park. You will find a trail intersection and a road crossing here. Continue going straight, unless you need the restrooms located at the pavilions.

You'll find another side trail to your left 0.3 miles from the pavilions, when you reach Jones Maltsberger Road on your left. Stay on the main trail to the right. The trail skirts the edge of the park, and a driving range is on your left, so keep an eye out for stray balls until you're safely past it. You'll be out of range when you reach the first low-water crossing after the driving range. You'll notice several houses on the left of the trail as you continue, and you'll reach a second low-water crossing. After this crossing, the baseball fields are again visible, and a side trail is to the left. This is the same side trail you passed at the beginning of the hike. Stay to the right, where you'll cross the road and walk into the pavilion area you passed earlier. A bulletin board with a map of the trail is the only map available. Once you've made use of any of the facilities you need, continue past the pavilions, where you'll reach a turnoff to the right. Take the right.

Astoundingly, considering no official trailhead is here, at 2 miles into the hike, you'll reach an obelisk-style marker that reads 2 miles. Just past this marker, a spur is to the right—continue going straight. You'll then reach another low-water crossing, and as you come up the rise, you'll see a police substation on your right. The creek bed you just crossed will be visible to your left but inaccessible. Hidden in the thick trees along the trail is a barbed-wire fence, so keep a close eye on your pets and children.

You'll reach another intersection at about 2.5 miles into the hike. A trail is to the left, and this is the one you want to take. Both trails lead back to where you parked; this one just offers a little more scenery. The number of deer seen in this park is impressive, considering its location inside the city limits. Keep a keen eye on the trees, and you should see plenty. You'll reach another fork by the park road. This time, take the right fork across the road.

You'll begin skirting several small and secluded picnic areas, and the bird and small mammal population is thickest here, as they scamper around looking for leftovers. After almost 0.5 miles of picnic areas, you'll reach a T-intersection. Take the right, as this is the trail on which you began, and your car is just across the road. You'll notice that the trail keeps going across the road—this is the link-up from the fork near the police station.

NEARBY ACTIVITIES

The park offers picnic facilities aplenty, as well as ball fields and a dog park.

49 MEDINA RIVER NATURAL AREA LOOP

KEY AT-A-GLANCE INFORMATION

LENGTH: 2.3 miles

CONFIGURATION: Loop

DIFFICULTY: Easy

SCENERY: Wooded river bottom, open upland

EXPOSURE: Mostly shaded

TRAFFIC: Moderate

TRAIL SURFACE: Concrete, natural surfaces

HIKING TIME: 1.2 hours

DRIVING DISTANCE: 15 miles from the Alamo

ACCESS: Daily, 7:30 a.m.–sunset; closed Christmas and New Year's Day; no fees

WHEELCHAIR ACCESS: Yes, along El Camino and Chaparral Trail

MAPS: sanaturalareas.org/cr/ crtrails.html

FACILITIES: Restrooms, water, picnicking at trailhead

CONTACT INFORMATION: (210) 207-8480; sanaturalareas.org/cr/ crindex.html

GPS TRAILHEAD COORDINATES

LATITUDE: 29° 15' 49.91"
LONGITUDE: 98° 34' 41.36"

IN BRIEF

This loop explores lush bottomland along the Medina River, where cypress and cottonwoods grow to mammoth proportions. The scenic Medina River adds to the beauty. The hike loops from the bottoms and joins the Chaparral Trail, a linear path that is part of the San Antonio greenways system, and then returns to the trailhead.

DESCRIPTION

If events had gone differently, what is now Medina River Natural Area would be underwater as a reservoir. Instead, we have the establishment of the 500-acre natural area, opened in 2005, which protects a bottomland corridor along the Medina River and also provides a venue for nature trails as well as one of San Antonio's linear greenways, the Chaparral Trail. The river bottoms contain some incredibly large cypress, cottonwood, and pecan trees that you have to see to believe. Sometimes in Central Texas we get used to seeing only smaller trees, but these bottomland giants will amaze. Much of the hike travels where you cannot only enjoy the big trees but also the Medina River as it flows to meet the San Antonio River.

Concrete trails spur away from the main trailhead near the park office and butterfly gardens. Look right for a concrete path leading

----

Directions

From Exit 49 on I-410 south of downtown San Antonio, take TX 16 south, Poteet Highway, for 4.2 miles to turn left into the natural area, just before the bridge over the Medina River. Follow the entrance road a short distance to the parking area.

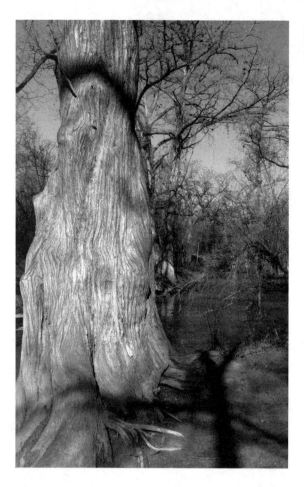

Gigantic flood-sculpted cypress trees line Rio Medina.

toward the river and fishing, the El Camino Trail. It descends by switchbacks to the Medina River and adjacent bottoms. Come to a large picnic pavilion and begin heading downstream along the waterway. At 0.3 miles reach a trail junction. Here, a concrete path continues right to dead-end at the river's edge. Go ahead and follow this to check out the Medina River up close. Admire the immense cypress trees lining the river. The hike continues on a gravel track, the Rio Medina Trail, bordered by hackberry and other hardwoods. At 0.4 miles a side trail leads right to a gigantic cypress. It would take multiple hikers to stretch their arms around it. Other spur trails lead to streamside fishing venues. At one time the Medina was known as the Catfish River.

The waterway sometimes flows quietly, and sometimes it gathers in noisy rapids. At 0.5 miles the Rio Medina Trail splits. Stay right with the path closest to the river, entering bona fide bottomland. Another spur trail leads down to a gravel bar along the stream, where you can access the river. The Medina River has its humble beginnings on the west side of Bandera County, where it gains water from springs emerging from the Balcones Escarpment. It continues following gravity's orders, entering Medina County, where the river is dammed as Medina Lake and Medina Diversion Reservoir before being freed again. The Medina next flows through Castroville and into Bexar County to meet the San Antonio River after a nearly 120-mile journey. The Medina's end is not far downstream from Medina River Natural Area. The narrow waterway flows beneath limestone bluffs and in other places simply cuts a channel through the soil, but it also has rocky sections. On this hike you will get a good look at the river. Paddlers ply the slender waterway, which offers Class I and Class II rocky rapids, but it is perhaps better known for its sharp turns that can spill novice boaters. Outfitters are located on sections of the river, primarily between the town of Medina and Medina Lake, upstream in Bandera County. Spring is the best time to float the river as it usually has ample water. Fall paddlers can enjoy autumn colors if there is adequate flow.

As you walk along the river, stop to admire the size of the cottonwoods, pecans, and other trees such as ash, willow, and vines that couldn't survive beyond these bottoms. Because this is bottomland, the trail can be muddy in places, especially after rains. Watch for deer or their tracks. At 1 mile the Nogales Trail leaves left. Keep along the Medina, observing bluffs across the river. Shortly turn away from the waterway, northbound. Cross channels that flow only during floods. At 1.4 miles turn right with the Oolmos Spur, while the Rio Medina Trail keeps forward in bottomland. Make a short but steep climb into another world—dry uplands where mesquite provides scant cover.

Meet the Chaparral Trail, also known as the Medina River Greenway, at 1.6 miles. Join a concrete greenway heading westerly toward the trailhead. Pass the other end of the Nogales Trail and a power line at 1.7 miles. The trail undulates and then meets a connector to the Rio Medina Trail at 1.9 miles. Stay right with the greenway, passing through a fence and coming to a pair of chimneys marking an old ranch site. The concrete track explores open terrain, an old ranch house, and a pond before returning to the trailhead at 2.3 miles.

NEARBY ACTIVITIES

Medina River Natural Area offers a group campground on the south side of the Medina River.

50 SAN ANTONIO BOTANICAL GARDENS TRAIL

GPS TRAILHEAD COORDINATES

LATITUDE: 29° 45' 80.83"
LONGITUDE: 98° 45' 82.78"

IN BRIEF

This educational jaunt located just north of downtown San Antonio offers exhibits of local and exotic plant life that serves the secondary purpose of attracting a wide variety of birdlife to the area.

DESCRIPTION

The San Antonio Botanical Gardens were opened in 1980 as a living museum to help educate people to the role that plants have in the environment. A popular spot for educational outings, this hike is a better way to learn about local flora than trying to identify plants and trees from books. Three simulated Texas ecological areas highlight the garden, as well as modern-looking, pyramid-shaped greenhouses.

The guest center, the Daniel Sullivan Carriage House, is listed in the National Register of Historic Places. Constructed in 1896, it was moved stone by stone from its original location downtown to its current location. In fact, almost all of the structures were brought from other places and have some historical value. The carriage house now contains the Carriage House Kitchen and the Garden Gate Gift Shop. This is where you pay the entry fee and enter the gardens.

Outside the carriage house, the path leads up a set of stairs (a ramp for wheelchairs and strollers lies beside the stairs). You'll see a plaque at the top of the stairs with a map of the park, the same map shown in the brochure.

Directions

From US 281 in San Antonio, exit on Hilde brand Avenue east. Turn right on New Braunfels Road, and then take a left on Funston. The garden is on the left.

N

0   125   250
feet

To
New Braunfels
Avenue

East Texas
Exhibit

East Texas Lake

Schumacher
House

Hill Country
Exhibit

Rose
Garden

building

South Texas
Exhibit

Auld House

Cactus and
Succulent Garden

Sullivan
Carriage House

P

Sunday
House

fountain

conservatory

Old Austin Road

To
New Braunfels
Avenue

Funston Place

Marney Road

800
750
700
650
600
550
500
450
400

FEET

0.25   0.5   0.75   1   1.1

MILES

A signpost with arrows points every which way. Head to the stairs in front of you to continue the hike. At the top of the stairs, you'll see a large natural canopy of vines and a fountain in a courtyard. Turn left on this side of the fountain to visit the Texas habitat areas.

The path forks and a ramp with handrails leads up a light incline. Follow the dirt path in front of you. Unlike the interpretive hikes in outlying parks, the botanical gardens have signs identifying all the different trees and plants. Shortly after the path are a set of stairs leading down into the conservatory and a path leading around a hill with a gazebo perched on top. At the next two trail junctions, continue straight. A stone wall is here, and a small aqueduct is to the left of the path. The path forks at nearly 0.5 miles; the flagstone path goes right, and the path you're on continues left and turns to dirt. The one-acre lake before you is indicative of those found in east Texas. A nearby gumball-type machine allows visitors to purchase food for the ducks that live by the lake. Where the trail Ts up, take the path right (toward the east Texas exhibit) to begin the first loop of the hike.

The path that encircles the lake turns to mulch and has a lush canopy that shades the trail. Immediately to the right stands a small palisade-adobe building. This south Texas exhibit area showcases the trees and shrubs found in the southern part of the state, such as mesquite, blackbrush, and ebony. Notice the roofs of the two buildings are made from native plants.

The trail continues under the canopy to the east Texas area. Pines, sweet gums, and magnolias stand out as you look over the lake to the left. On the right side of the trail stands a log cabin and accompanying storage shed, both relocated from a 95-acre farm in Park, Texas, that was flooded by a new reservoir. The display even includes a garden with tomato and pepper plants.

When the trail forks again, stay to the left, continuing around the lake. A sign pointing to the Hill Country display reminds you that you're on the right track. The plants here—such as mountain cedar and laurel—are native to the Texas Hill Country, and area residents should be familiar with the majority of them. You can also see the Schumacher House. Built in 1849 from wood, mud, and sand, the structure was relocated from Fredericksburg. The next building on the trail, the Auld House, though not original, was based on a cabin in Leakey and is available for rental. You will also find a patio, water fountain, and restrooms.

Past the Auld House are a couple of garden areas with flagstone sidewalks, and you can see the visitor center to the right and the gazebo to the left on top of its hill. As you stroll through the wildflower trail on the way to the aforementioned garden areas, notice the size of the Hill Country live oak standing on the trail. You'll also see ball moss on the branches of the tree. Continue on to the garden areas, and then turn left back toward the fountain you passed when you came in.

At this point you can return to the carriage house or turn left and go to the Lucille Halsell Conservatory. These modern-looking greenhouses hold exhibits of European plants and flowers and trees from South America and Asia. The climate-controlled greenhouses offer an area in which to cool off on a warm afternoon and probably hold any plants you expected to see but didn't find in other areas.

SAN ANTONIO MISSION TRAIL 51

IN BRIEF

Stroll between and visit two historic missions along the historic and surprisingly lush San Antonio Mission Trail.

DESCRIPTION

San Antonio Missions National Historic Park consists of a chain of four missions along the San Antonio River—San José, San Juan, Espada, and Concepción. These structures, in conjunction with the Alamo, form the oldest chain of Catholic missions in North America. Originally lured here by rumors of wealth and the encroaching French from Louisiana, Spaniards established these missions in east Texas hoping to take advantage of local riches. Failing this, they set about converting the locals to Catholicism.

The first mission built in the area served as a waypoint between the missions in Louisiana–east Texas and New Spain (Mexico). This was Mission San Antonio de Valero, later known as the Alamo. Two years later, in 1720, Fray Antonio Margil de Jesús established a second mission, San José, for the purpose of converting the native Coahuiltecan tribes. In the meantime, the east Texas missions failed; three of these missions were relocated to the San Antonio area. The missions soon became not only religious centers but also cultural and economic centers, complete with fortified walls, farms with an irrigation system, and herds of sheep and cattle. Though considered historical sites, the missions are still active worship centers.

Directions ——————————————————➤

From I-35 exit at East Southcross Boulevard. Proceed west on Southcross to Roosevelt Avenue. Turn left and proceed south on Roosevelt until it intersects with Napier Avenue. Turn left. The visitor center is on your left.

KEY AT-A-GLANCE INFORMATION

LENGTH: 6 miles

CONFIGURATION: Out-and-back

DIFFICULTY: Very easy

SCENERY: Historic Spanish missions, San Antonio River

EXPOSURE: Open

TRAFFIC: Moderate–heavy

TRAIL SURFACE: Asphalt

HIKING TIME: Walking time is about 1.5 hours, but allow extra time to explore the missions

DRIVING DISTANCE: 82 miles from the state capitol

ACCESS: Daily, 9 a.m.–5 p.m.; closed Thanksgiving, Christmas, and New Year's Day; no fees or permits

WHEELCHAIR ACCESS: Yes

MAPS: nps.gov/saan

FACILITIES: Restrooms, gift shop, and picnic areas with barbecue pits

CONTACT INFORMATION: (210) 932-1001; nps.gov/saan

GPS TRAILHEAD COORDINATES

LATITUDE: 29° 36' 43.89"
LONGITUDE: 98° 48' 03.89"

51 San Antonio Mission Trail

N   0   0.25   0.5
mile

37

Mission Road

536

Padre Drive

122

New Braunfels Avenue

PYTEL PARK

Mission San José

PADRE PARK

San Antonio River

visitor center

To 35

13   S.W. Military Dr.

Harding Boulevard

13

March Avenue

J.F.K. MEMORIAL

S. Presa Street

Old Corpus Christi Hwy.

STINSON PARK

Roosevelt Avenue

Cadmus Street

Mission Road

ESPADA PARK

122

BELLAIRE PARK

Ashley Road

Ashley Road

Mission San Juan

Rilling Road

SAN ANTONIO MISSIONS NATIONAL HISTORICAL PARK

536

410 281

700
650
600
550
500
450
400
350
300

FEET

0.5   1   1.5   2   2.5   3

MILES

The park service asks that you respect services and parish staff.

The trail now exists between Mission Concepción to Mission Espada, though the National Park Service plans to complete a trail from the Alamo south to the Mission Espada. Currently, you can travel roads to the Alamo. The visitor center and park headquarters are located at Mission San José, where this hike begins.

Before starting your hike, explore the remains of the old mission at a leisurely pace. The size of Mission San José led to its being known as the "queen of the missions." The center of village life and source of its defense, the mission's large walls helped resident Native Americans fend off attacks by Apache and Comanche tribes.

The beginning of the hike is very open. The asphalt trail is officially known as the Mission Hike and Bike Trail but is commonly referred to as the Mission Trail. With the exception of the length, there is no reason why children couldn't enjoy this trail, and a stroller would be easy to push along. The trail starts at the visitor center and heads south across the parking lot area, reaching Padre Drive. Turn right and follow the trail as it parallels the road and passes a fenced-in field where sheep are still kept today.

Soon after the sheep enclosure, the trail widens and you'll arrive at the first of four footbridges; another lies just ahead. The path reaches the San Antonio River at just over 0.5 miles and continues beside it. The wide path continues south and reaches a small parking area known as Padre Park at 1.4 miles.

Pass under Military Drive and then arrive at Espada Park 1.8 miles into the trail, where you'll find parking spaces, picnic tables, and grills set up for public use. A short way south of the park, the path separates from the road, which crosses the river at Espada Dam, and continues along the west bank of the river.

The trail is wide and in very good shape, and it's more pleasant for leaving the traffic behind, albeit briefly. Shortly after leaving the road you'll come to a third footbridge, at which point the trail stands about 40 feet above the river at normal levels. As you walk along this section, look to the right and you can see portions of the Acequia de Espada, the remains of a gravity-flow ditch system. These *acequias* remain as part of a larger system of dams and aqueducts that were used to irrigate the missions' fields for agricultural use. Espada Dam still diverts water into the Acequia Madre, or "mother ditch," which is carried over Sixmile Creek by the oldest Spanish aqueduct in North America, the Espada Aqueduct. This system still provides water to nearby farms.

Continuing southward, you'll reach a stone embankment on your right that prevents further erosion and, shortly thereafter, the fourth and final footbridge crosses another feeder creek. At 2.6 miles the trail joins Ashley Road. Turn left onto the road and keep an eye out for approaching traffic. Just across the river, you can turn right and walk into the parking lot for the San Juan mission.

Mission San Juan Capistrano was originally established as San José de los Nazonis in east Texas. Relocated to this spot in 1731, it oversaw a rich agricultural area and orchards that supported not only the mission but also the nearby settlements and presidio. Take the time to explore the old building before heading back up the trail to Mission San José.

North of San Antonio (Hikes 52-60)

N

0   7.5   15
miles

NORTH OF
SAN ANTONIO

52 BAR-O RANCH LOOP

KEY AT-A-GLANCE INFORMATION

LENGTH: 4.4 miles

CONFIGURATION: Loop

DIFFICULTY: Moderate

SCENERY: Wide creek valley, cedar woods

EXPOSURE: Mostly open

TRAFFIC: Moderate

TRAIL SURFACE: Dirt, rocks

HIKING TIME: 2.75 hours

DRIVING DISTANCE: 52 miles from the Alamo

ACCESS: Daily, 8 a.m.–10 p.m.; closed during public hunts; $6 day-use fee/person over age 13

WHEELCHAIR ACCESS: No

MAPS: tpwd.state.tx.us/ publications

FACILITIES: Untreated water, privy at park headquarters

CONTACT INFORMATION: (830) 796-4413; tpwd.state.tx.us/spdest/ findadest/parks/hill_country

GPS TRAILHEAD COORDINATES

LATITUDE: 29° 62' 73.06"
LONGITUDE: 99° 17' 80.56"

IN BRIEF

This hike travels the lower West Verde Creek Valley at Hill Country State Natural Area. Start at the park headquarters and make a wide loop around the old Bar-O Ranch. Along the way you'll see waterfalls, hillside cedar forests, old pastureland, and the valley of West Verde Creek.

DESCRIPTION

This hike traverses the lower elevations of Hill Country State Natural Area, staying in the vicinity of the old Bar-O Ranch main house. The main ranch house was built in 1916 and is used today by the Hill Country State Natural Area park manager. This is cattle country, and you will see relics from the ranch days. This hike through ranching history is in an appealing natural setting. You'll come to a small falls shortly after the trailhead and then climb into a hillside cedar forest, where the views open. Dip back down to West Verde Creek, where you'll pass the old Chapa House before ascending along West Verde Creek. Comanche Bluffs tower over the stream, which makes another drop at Chaquita Falls.

Park near the mailbox at park headquarters and then walk down the park road north, away from the mailbox and past the park office. Look right for Trail #2, Bar-O Pasture

Directions

From San Antonio take TX 16 to Bandera. In Bandera, turn left on TX 173 south, following it for one mile to FR 1077. Turn right onto FR 1077 and follow it for 10 miles to the park, where the road turns to dirt. Turn right into the park, crossing West Verde Creek, and then turn right into the parking area near the park headquarters.

N

0   0.2   0.4
mile

HILL COUNTRY
STATE NATURAL AREA

West Verde Creek

private road

9B

9B

Comanche Bluff
Camp Area

8B

8

Chapa's Group
Camp Area

chemical
toilet

Chaquita Falls
Camp Area

9C

9A

9

9

9

2B

To
Bandera

RR 1017

2C

West Verde Creek

2

2C

2B

2B

8A

W. Verde
Camp Area

8

8

house

park
headquarters

chemical
toilet

P

Bar-O
Camp Area

Bandera Creek Road

To
Tarpley
and FM 462

CR 131

chemical
toilet

5A

7

7

6

P

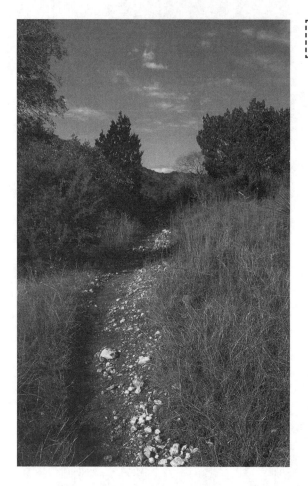

Trail. Take Trail #2 and follow it a bit before it splits. Stay right, passing through a fence, and then keep along a fence line to reach another junction. Trail #2B leaves left. Stay right, heading downstream along West Verde Creek, and pass a dam on the creek. You are heading toward the old two-story ranch house. At almost 0.5 miles, the trail crosses West Verde Creek just before reaching the house. Falls drop both above and below the crossing. The low flow of West Verde Creek makes the cascades less spectacular than they would be in more high-precipitation locations.

Pass an old barn before reaching an intersection at just over 0.5 miles. Trail #2C keeps forward. Trail #2B goes left and right. Turn right on Trail #2B to cross the county road heading toward Bandera. Immediately ascend a cedar-studded hill. The hills across West Verde Creek stand tall in the distance. The path is rocky in places. More good views open as you descend to reach a metal barn and Trail #9, Pasture Loop Trail. Veer left here onto a doubletrack path to cross a fence at 1.3 miles. Turn left here onto Trail #9A, Cedar Trail. Begin shadowing the cedar post and wire fence marking the park boundary. Ride the fence line like an old Texas cowpoke checking for breaches. The narrow path curves with the boundary fence ahead and enters dense woods near the dam of an old pond.

The trail opens up to a hillside beyond the dam. Hill Country State Natural Area stands before you to the west. At 2.6 miles intersect Trail #9. Keep right here, heading downhill. Shortly Trail #9B, Eagle Trail, leaves left. This is a good side trip if you want to extend the loop. Dip to cross another pond dam and reach the fertile ground of an open field. The backside of Chapa House lies ahead. Reach Chapa House at 3.2 miles. This is another part of the former ranch complex.

Cross the park road and head for the low-water bridge spanning West Verde Creek. Directly beside West Verde Creek is Trail #8A, Chaquita Falls Trail. Head upstream along West Verde Creek on Chaquita Falls Trail. The two deep pools are popular fishing and swimming holes. The Comanche Bluffs Camping Area is just to the right of the trail. The actual Comanche Bluffs are to the left of the stream. Cross the stream ahead at 3.4 miles. A simple rock-hop is in order, except during floods, when you wouldn't be on the trail at all. Enter a live oak cathedral before emerging just above Chaquita Falls. This wide, low-flow water feature slips over a rock slab into a pool. The Chaquita Falls Camp Area is nearby on this side of the stream.

A mix of grass and trees lies ahead, backed by a tall bluff. At 4.1 miles intersect the Hightower Trail. Turn right here and cruise through mixed woods and open country to reach the park headquarters trailhead.

53   CIBOLO NATURE CENTER HIKE

KEY AT-A-GLANCE INFORMATION

LENGTH: 2.9 miles

CONFIGURATION: Irregular

DIFFICULTY: Easy

SCENERY: Wetlands, tall grass, Cibolo Creek, surrounding woodlands

EXPOSURE: Very sunny–very shady

TRAFFIC: Moderate

TRAIL SURFACE: Grass, dirt, boardwalk

HIKING TIME: 1.5 hours

DRIVING DISTANCE: 33 miles from the Alamo

ACCESS: Daily, 8 a.m.–sunset; no fees, but donations welcome

WHEELCHAIR ACCESS: Yes, in some sections

MAPS: cibolo.org/visitors

FACILITIES: Restrooms and picnic tables; beverages and gifts available in the visitor center

CONTACT INFORMATION: (830) 249-4616; cibolo.org

GPS TRAILHEAD COORDINATES

LATITUDE: 29° 78' 51.11"
LONGITUDE: 98° 71' 31.94"

IN BRIEF

This is a wonderful area and an easy hike where families can learn about the various ecosystems represented in the preserve, located on the outskirts of Boerne. A wetland boardwalk, tallgrass prairie, and dinosaur tracks will hold the interest of even the youngest hikers.

DESCRIPTION

Nestled on the east side of Boerne, the 100-acre Cibolo Nature Center attracts thousands of visitors each year. This nature preserve and environmental learning center contain numerous exhibits that educate hikers and visitors about the area's distinct ecosystems. Inside the visitor center are any number of informative pamphlets, including lists of birds typically found in the area as well as some nature books on Texas.

The trailhead is located at a pavilion north of the visitor center, where you will also find restrooms. The three plaques here display a map of the trail system, give information on the ecological areas, and explain the dinosaur tracks located 80 feet up the trail.

Continue past the plaques to reach the tracks, which are actually replicas of prints uncovered at the Boerne Lake spillway in June 1997 after a flood. The spillway is inaccessible to the public, so Peggy Maceo, an Austin-area artist, made these exact copies to be placed here for public view. Molds were made of the

----

Directions

From Exit 542 on I-10, take US 87 to Boerne. From Boerne, take TX 46 east toward Boerne City Park; turn right on City Park Road. Cibolo Nature Center is on the right and is marked by a sign at its gate.

original prints and then cast in concrete and arranged to replicate the spillway site. The dinosaur that made these prints is identified as the carnivore Acrocanthosaurus and has been found in other parts of the state, including the famous Glenn Rose formation in central Texas. The limestone of Boerne Lake is part of this same formation.

Just past the tracks you'll reach a wooden bridge spanning a creek bed and then a trail junction, bench, and accompanying directional signs. You'll head left to the Prairie and Creek trails in a bit, but meanwhile head right along the Marsh Loop. The surrounding area is part of the replicated tallgrass prairie, with numerous birdhouses and nesting boxes on the property. Look closely and you'll see a bat house on the right. The trail forks at 0.2 miles. Stay right and return from the left.

Follow the boardwalk, which was built by students from the local high school, through the marsh. Set on short pilings, the walkway carries you right into the middle of the marsh for an up-close look. A short distance ahead, the boardwalk expands into a wider deck area, where a bench is set up overlooking the largest part of the pool. The water here is crystal clear. Small fish and insects swim on and below its surface. The marsh area is also home to several bird species, including cattle egret, redwing blackbirds, and kingfishers. A smaller deck amid the tall grass lies just beyond this point.

The boardwalk ends at the edge of the Boerne City Park. The trail turns to the left and loops back into the preserve, along the edge of the marsh. Another bench on the trail allows you to observe the marsh from outside of it. Just beyond this, the loop closes and the trail returns to the junction, where you'll see a marker designating the area as the Hilmar-Bergman Historical Prairie. This time follow the directional signs to the Prairie Loop Trail. Just before you reach a playground area and covered kiosk, you'll come to a trail intersection to the left. Take this trail to hike down toward the creek. The path soon crosses a dirt road where a sign warns drivers of hikers in the area. Cross the road and continue down the trail.

The trail joins Cibolo Creek, marked on the trail map as The Narrows. As you walk beside the creek, you'll notice how clear the water is. The creek area is part of the Texas Watch Stream Monitoring program and is checked for quality regularly as a critical source of recharge for the Edwards Aquifer. Anglers are occasionally seen here hoping to hook into one of the creek's bass or catfish that can easily be seen from some of the higher points on the trail. Snapping turtles also make their homes here.

The tall cypress trees provide ample shade for this part of the hike, which narrows considerably. After walking about 0.2 miles into the Cypress Trail, you'll encounter an earthen staircase leading away from the creek. Take these stairs, which will join you with the Woodland Loop Trail. Turn right onto the trail.

The environment here could not differ more from the tallgrass prairie you walked through earlier. Oaks and junipers create a dense canopy over this trail, which follows the creek bluff before looping back north. Deer, rabbits, and numerous birds make their home in the cover provided by the trees, and the American beauty bush and Mexican buckeye stay on the ground. Keep an ear open for rustling in the brush, and you might catch a glimpse of the nine-banded armadillo.

As the trail winds through woodlands, it meets with a high electric fence 1.2 miles into the hike. This fence serves to keep predators out of the ranch across from it. A bench faces the fence, offering views of birds and wildlife on the other side.

Not far past the bench, the path splits. Take the trail to the left, which leads back to the creek.

You'll soon return to the earthen stairs leading back down to the creek. Walk down and turn right to backtrack toward the kiosk area and the remainder of the Prairie Loop. When you reach the road you crossed before (1.8 miles), turn left onto it and hike past the picnic tables to your left. This section is the Cypress Trail on the map.

Continue hiking along the river until you reach the edge of the city park's soccer fields at 2.3 miles. Turn to the right. Numerous trees here are protected by fencing, and the map designates the area as the Tree of Life Arboretum. At nearly 2.5 miles you'll see tennis courts on your left. Directly to your right is the beginning of another trail. This leads through the grassland prairie and back to the visitor center. Take this trail. As you walk along with the tall grass on both sides, look and listen for rattlesnakes and rabbits coming in and out of the thick prairie. At 2.8 miles the trail rejoins the Prairie Loop Trail, which leads left to the pavilion. Turn left here and head back that way and then take the right, which leads to the small wooden bridge and the visitor center, where you can stop in and visit with the staff, pick up something cold to drink, and maybe make a contribution to their ongoing project.

NEARBY ACTIVITIES

The nature center offers numerous continual outreach programs and is available for rental.

54 GUADALUPE RIVER STATE PARK LOOP

KEY AT-A-GLANCE INFORMATION

LENGTH: 2.8 miles

CONFIGURATION: Loop

DIFFICULTY: Easy–moderate

SCENERY: Open and wooded hills, river bluff

EXPOSURE: Mostly open

TRAFFIC: Moderate, busy on weekends

TRAIL SURFACE: Natural surfaces

HIKING TIME: 1.5 hours

DRIVING DISTANCE: 38 miles from the Alamo

ACCESS: Daily, 8 a.m.–10 p.m.; $7 entrance fee/person over age 13

WHEELCHAIR ACCESS: No

MAPS: tpwd.state.tx.us/ publications

FACILITIES: Restrooms, picnicking, and camping at park; none at trailhead

CONTACT INFORMATION: (830) 438-2656; tpwd.state.tx.us/spdest/ findadest/parks/guadalupe_river

GPS TRAILHEAD COORDINATES

LATITUDE: 29° 51' 37.91"
LONGITUDE: 98° 29' 59.62"

IN BRIEF

This state park, a long-time favorite of central Texans, has added a series of multiuse loop trails that travel through the heart of the park and along bluffs above the Guadalupe River, where views await from tall river bluffs.

DESCRIPTION

Hikers will be glad to know that more trail mileage has been added to this destination. A popular spot for all types of outdoor enthusiasts, Guadalupe River State Park has managed to maintain its rugged beauty in spite of the large number of visitors that it receives. Located on a stretch of the Guadalupe River, the park includes 4 miles of river frontage, multiple campsites, and day-use areas. During the summer months it is almost sure to be full to capacity because of the cold waters of the river. The best times to visit during this season would be early in the week and as early in the morning as possible. Most park visitors will be on the river, and though the multiple-use trails are near the Guadalupe, they are high on a bluff, minimizing interaction with the potentially busy—but beautiful— riverside area.

The loop trails travel uplands comprising wooded grassy locale and ever-present rocks. Trails are quite stony, though dirt finds its place. The trail system is open to mountain bikers and equestrians, though the equestrians

---

Directions

From US 281 north of San Antonio near Bulverde, take TX 46 west for 4 miles to Park Road 31. Turn right on Park Road 31 and follow it 3 miles to enter the park. Once beyond the entrance station, continue 4.5 miles to the trailhead on your left.

N

0   0.1   0.2
mile

GUADALUPE RIVER
STATE PARK

Guadalupe River

Guadalupe River

Cedar Sage
Camp Area

Loop 3

Guadalupe River State Park Road

Park Road 31

P

Loop 2

Loop 4

P

To 46

FEET						
1,400						
1,350						
1,300						
1,250						
1,200						
1,150						
1,100						
1,050						
1,000	0.5	1	1.5	2	2.5	2.8

MILES

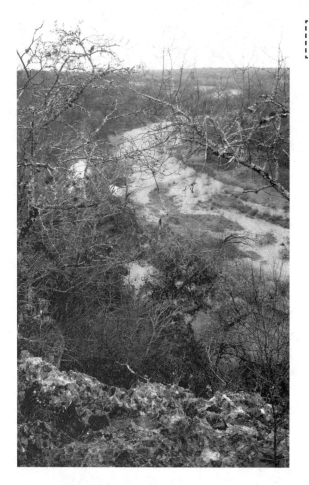

Blufftop view of the Guadalupe River

have their own separate trailhead near the park entrance station.

From the main trailhead beyond the entrance station, head north and join a doubletrack path, Loop 2, traveling amid scattered oaks and juniper with occasional cacti. Before long you pass the first of many square hunting blinds, small buildings that resemble phone booths. Shootists use these seasonally during winter, when public hunts are allowed in the park. These hunts occur to keep the native white-tailed deer population controlled, as well as to eliminate exotic species such as wild hogs and axis deer, an Asian native. Consider entering a blind yourself to perhaps observe critters roaming this park. Contact the park about hunts should you decide to hike here during December or January. At 0.2 miles pass under a transmission line and then begin a downgrade. At 0.4 miles tunnel through a live oak copse, where widespread branches shade the path. The trail then circles around the remains of an old pond before reaching a trail junction at 0.6 miles. Turn left here, joining Loop 3. Keep north toward the Guadalupe River in a hodgepodge of oak groves and stony meadows. A fence delineating the park boundary stands to your left.

Come alongside a bluff above the Guadalupe River at 1 mile. The rocky track curves right, keeping the bluff and the river to your left. You are heading downstream. The waterway flows 100-plus feet below. Occasional spur paths lead to partially wooded dark outcrops that avail views of the bending Guadalupe. Cypress trees find their place while gravel gathers in the shallows. In still other places fallen boulders stand against the flow. At normal flows the river will display an aquamarine color. Rapids add an audio component to the scenery. The limestone bluffs have been eroded by centuries of flowing water. Hawks and buzzards are constantly soaring along its edges. Small swallows nest in holes in the bluff. An abandoned ranch stands across the water.

At 1.3 miles reach a trail junction near a stock tank. A shaded picnic table beckons. Here a trail keeps forward to reach the Cedar Sage Camping Area, emerging between campsites #33 and #34. Loop 3 turns right here, away from the Guadalupe River, and begins a gentle ascent toward the main park road. Pass a second spur to the campground as you wander amid grassy glens and dense woodlands. Turn sharply westerly at 1.6 miles to meet a live oak grove with branches draped in moss and epiphytes. At 2 miles a resting bench avails a view of Texas Hill Country. At 2.2 miles reach a trail junction. Stay left here, rejoining Loop 2 as it heads south. Moderately ascend to reach Park Road 31 at 2.4 miles. Walk along the park road shoulder, making your way back to the main trailhead, completing the loop. You can extend your hike by crossing Park Road 31 and tackling Loop 4.

NEARBY ACTIVITIES

Mountain View Park has shaded picnic facilities, a short hard-surface trail, and playgrounds.

55 GUADALUPE RIVER TRAIL

KEY AT-A-GLANCE INFORMATION

LENGTH: 1 mile

CONFIGURATION: Out-and-back

DIFFICULTY: Moderate

SCENERY: Lush woods, Guadalupe River

EXPOSURE: Shady

TRAFFIC: Light

TRAIL SURFACE: Gravel, dirt, roots

HIKING TIME: 30 minutes

DRIVING DISTANCE: 50 miles from the Alamo

ACCESS: Daily, 7 a.m.–10 p.m.; no fees or permits

WHEELCHAIR ACCESS: Yes, on short path to nearby fishing pier

MAPS: None

FACILITIES: None

CONTACT INFORMATION: (830) 964-3341; swf-wc.usace.army.mil/canyon

GPS TRAILHEAD COORDINATES

LATITUDE: 29° 86' 91.39"
LONGITUDE: 98° 19' 21.94"

IN BRIEF

The premier spot for fly fishermen throughout the state, this isolated trail located near Canyon Lake Tailrace also offers hikers a quiet reprieve from the busier parks in summer.

DESCRIPTION

Water from the Guadalupe River exits Canyon Lake Dam just upstream from here and offers the coldest year-round water in the state. Anglers from all over the state know it as the only place where rainbow trout exist throughout the year. Just downriver, inner tube, kayak, and canoe enthusiasts begin a traditional spring and summer float trip that can lead hard-core floaters all the way to New Braunfels.

River recreation here is commonly thought of as anything but tranquil. However, this hidden trail begins and ends before the sometimes-rowdy floaters begin their trek. For birders, anglers, and nature watchers, it is a small oasis of tranquility located in one of the busiest summertime getaway spots in the state.

A short hike through the thick bottoms of the river, this trail offers birders a chance to see the endangered black-capped vireo playing in the tall tops of the trees. Another draw is the population of wading birds that one would normally observe on the lakes or near the coast. Shallow pools and eddies here create a natural environment for birds such as sandpipers,

Directions

From I-35 South take FM 306 west to South Access Road. Turn left on South Access Road and look on the left for the park entrance. There are two parking areas. Turn into the second parking lot. A large sign at the end designates the beginning of the trail.

egrets, and herons to probe for a meal or rest in this lush watershed.

The trail begins by descending a short earthen staircase at the end of the parking lot. A wooden bridge is located almost immediately after the stairs, and a second one appears within 500 feet. The first half of the trail is very well kept, with wood guards keeping the gravel of the trail even and easy to traverse. The river is barely visible through the dense trees, but the sounds of the water are always present. The thick plants and wildflowers are natural attractants for a variety of butterflies in the spring and summer. The canopy and the cool air coming off the river keep this hike relatively cool throughout the year. Numerous spurs lead to the river, where it is generally shallow enough to wade. Anglers use these trails to get to prime fishing spots.

You'll encounter a bench and scenic river overlook 0.2 miles into the trail, where you can watch the wading birds and anglers play in the river. Even if you aren't an angler, the display put on by a skilled fly fisherman can be entrancing. The hypnotic rhythms used to deftly place the delicate lures within striking distance of hungry trout will entrance most observers, who quickly learn that the sport has more to do with casting than catching fish. It is an art form that one must observe to truly appreciate, and this is a great location to see it.

The trail continues at its current state for another tenth of a mile until it reaches a set of wood-and-earth stairs leading downward, where it narrows into a simple dirt path. If you're wearing shorts, you might want to consider turning back at this point. The thick ground cover hugs the trail for the remainder of the hike.

At this point the habitat becomes very inviting to black-capped vireos. Listen for their singing and scan the treetops for motion. The tiny, reclusive birds can be seen hanging from the branches, darting back and forth between the trees. You'll have to be very still and quiet to get a good look at this endangered bird. They offer their songs, however, to even the nosiest of passersby.

The attraction of the water and surrounding woods is irresistible to numerous small mammals. Squirrels are abundant both in the trees and on the ground, and nutria can be heard rummaging in the weeds and along the bank. Looking like a cross between a beaver and a big rat, the herbivorous nutria can be somewhat alarming the first time you see one. They are usually harmless and want nothing to do with people, so they'll insist you watch them from a distance. Most of the small holes you see along this and other river trails in the area are made by them rooting for food.

The trail continues to push into the thick woodland until you reach a point where you simply can't go any farther—a little more than 0.5 miles from the trailhead. Not far off the trail is a wetlands restoration habitat. This trail is under a constant state of improvement; it will someday connect with the wetlands viewing area. Maintained by the U.S. Army Corps of Engineers, both areas would make a great wild attraction in this otherwise busy area. Talk continues of extending this trail; consider calling the corps and urging them to extend the path.

As you return, take the time to observe the damage that floods can do to the landscape. Numerous large trees lay on their sides, victims of raging floods.

HIGHTOWER TRAIL HIKE 56

IN BRIEF

Hill Country State Natural Area is the setting for this fine loop. Work away from park headquarters up to high points with views. Circle around former ranch country before descending to West Verde Creek, where great views await at Comanche Bluffs. Finally pass an old ranch homestead and then follow the creek past Chaquita Falls, a small cascade on West Verde Creek.

DESCRIPTION

This is one of my favorite hikes in central Texas. It shows off the Hill Country at its finest, passing across both forested and open peaks where you can look out on wildlands. At the same time it visits old ranch relics, for the Hill Country is ranch country if nothing else. The water feature of West Verde Creek adds contrast to the loop—you overlook the watercourse from Comanche Bluffs before dropping creekside to view Chaquita Falls.

The Hightower Trail begins near the mailbox near the park headquarters. Trails at Hill Country State Natural Area are marked with numbered plastic posts. Leave the headquarters area on Trail #8, Hightower Trail. Shortly pass through a break in an old fence.

Directions

From San Antonio take TX 16 to Bandera. In Bandera turn left on TX 173 south, following 173 for 1 mile to FR 1077. Turn right onto FR 1077 and follow it 10 miles to the park, where the road turns to dirt. Turn right in the park, crossing West Verde Creek, and then turn right again into the park headquarters. Park near the headquarters or across the road near the Bar-O Ranch Camping Area.

KEY AT-A-GLANCE INFORMATION

LENGTH: 4.3 miles

CONFIGURATION: Loop

DIFFICULTY: Moderate–difficult

SCENERY: Wooded hills, creek

EXPOSURE: Partly shady

TRAFFIC: Moderate, busy on spring and fall weekends

TRAIL SURFACE: Rocks aplenty, dirt

HIKING TIME: 2.75 hours

DRIVING DISTANCE: 52 miles from the Alamo

ACCESS: Daily, 8 a.m.–10 p.m.; closed during public hunts; $6 day-use fee/person over age 13

WHEELCHAIR ACCESS: No

MAPS: tpwd.state.tx.us/publications

FACILITIES: Untreated water and privy near park office

CONTACT INFORMATION: (830) 796-4413; tpwd.state.tx.us/spdest/findadest/parks/hill_country

GPS TRAILHEAD COORDINATES

LATITUDE: 29° 62' 73.06"
LONGITUDE: 99° 17' 80.56"

Overlooking West Verde Creek

At 0.3 miles the Hightower Trail stays forward with a doubletrack path, whereas Trail #8A, the Chaquita Falls Trail, splits to the left. The Chaquita Falls Trail is part of your return route.

Begin to ascend a partly wooded hill. Views open to your west atop the hill, and live oaks grow plentifully up here. The Hightower Trail drifts through live oak groves. At almost 1 mile, the path bisects an old ranch gate near a tin shed. Cut through a second gate and descend into a grassy swale before climbing toward a small transmission line. Turn left here to top a second hill. The trail is very rocky on the downgrade. Boulders, pebbles, and stones of every size cover the trail. Dip to an old watering hole at 1.7 miles. A concrete basin, shed, and salt lick are hereabouts.

The Hightower Trail now undulates northerly through hills. Views open up, and the solitude is palpable. No sounds of trucks rumbling in the distance can be heard here. Begin to follow a rocky wash before crossing it to make a gap in the ridgeline to your left. Descend from the gap toward West Verde Creek on a doubletrack path. Look for a side trail leading left at 2.7 miles. This trail, the Comanche Bluffs Trail, is easily missed. This path leads 0.1 mile left to bluffs overlooking West Verde Creek. The rock bluffs shadow the clear pools of the watercourse. Comanche Bluffs Camp Area is below in the grove of live oak trees. You can also see the low-water bridge downstream on the creek, which you will be crossing shortly.

Backtrack and resume descending to a private ranch road. Turn left here and cross the low-water bridge. The Chapa House is to the right of the bridge. The route turns left just after the low-water bridge, now as the Chaquita Falls Trail. Begin to cruise along West Verde Creek. Look for turtles sunning on logs and rocks and for bream beneath the water. Comanche Bluffs Camping Area is just to

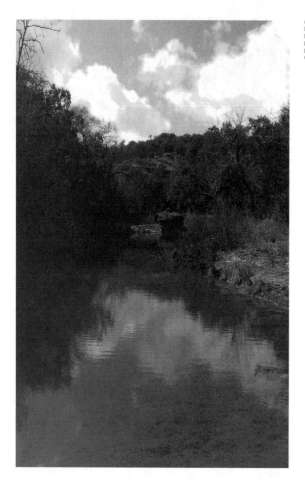

Clear water drains Texas Hill Country.

the right of the trail. Cross the stream ahead at 3.3 miles, a task that should be easy in times of normal flow. Stroll beneath live oaks before you climb out just above Chaquita Falls, a wide cascade that drops 4 or 5 feet into a pool. The Chaquita Falls Camp Area is nearby on this side of the stream.

A mix of grass and trees lies ahead. A tall bluff to the left is visible from open areas. To your right you can see the old Bar-O Ranch homesite, built in 1916. At 4 miles you'll intersect High-tower Trail. Turn right here and backtrack 0.3 miles to the trailhead.

NEARBY ACTIVITIES

Hill Country State Natural Area offers walk-in tent camping, backpacking, bicycling, horseback riding, and fishing.

HILL COUNTRY AND CANYON TREK

IN BRIEF

This challenging hike traverses the highs and lows of Hill Country State Natural Area. You'll begin along the creek bottoms of a wide valley and then climb into some bona fide Hill Country after a lung-buster climb. Dip down to a backcountry campsite before roaming into Cougar Canyon, where views await you. From here, a long downgrade eases the pain of the trek's end.

DESCRIPTION

This is one of the best hikes in the entire Hill Country region. It explores all the different environments Hill Country State Natural Area offers. Much of the hike offers a truly wild feel, and if you are up to the task, two backpack campsites are on the way. Leave the main day-use trailhead at the end of public vehicular access, and begin to walk down the closed park road north, away from the park office, up the West Verde Creek Valley.

At 0.1 mile, turn right onto Trail #6, Spring Branch Trail. The trails at Hill Country State Natural Area are numbered on plastic posts in the field and have corresponding names. All trails in the park are open to hikers, bikers, and equestrians. Descend through broken woods and pasture to shortly meet Trail

KEY AT-A-GLANCE INFORMATION

LENGTH: 7.8 miles

CONFIGURATION: Loop

DIFFICULTY: Difficult

SCENERY: Wooded and open hills, canyons, creek bottomland

EXPOSURE: Mostly open

TRAFFIC: Moderate—potentially busy on nice spring and fall weekends

TRAIL SURFACE: Dirt, rocks

HIKING TIME: 5.5 hours

DRIVING DISTANCE: 52 miles from the Alamo

ACCESS: Daily, 8 a.m.–10 p.m.; closed during public hunts; $6 day-use fee/person over age 13

WHEELCHAIR ACCESS: No

MAPS: tpwd.state.tx.us/publications

FACILITIES: Untreated water and privy near park office

CONTACT INFORMATION: (830) 796-4413; tpwd.state.tx.us/spdest/findadest/parks/hill_country

Directions

From San Antonio take TX 16 to Bandera. In Bandera turn left on TX 173 south, following 173 for 1 mile to FR 1077. Turn right onto FR 1077 and follow it 10 miles to the park, where the road turns to dirt. Turn right into the park, crossing West Verde Creek, and then turn right again, passing the park headquarters. Continue to the day-use parking area on your left.

GPS TRAILHEAD COORDINATES

LATITUDE: 29° 62' 73.06"
LONGITUDE: 99° 17' 80.56"

0   0.2   0.4
mile

CR 131

chemical toilet

5A

6

1A

To Tarpley and RM 462

2B

9

Twin Peaks

closed park road

5

5

2A

cattle guard

5

boarded house

4

4B

HILL COUNTRY STATE NATURAL AREA

3

West Verde Creek

Wilderness Camp Area

3A

3

4B

4B

Cougar Canyon

3B

3A

Butterfly Springs Camp Area

4A

Hermit's Shack Camp Area

FEET					
2,000					
1,900					
1,800					
1,700					
1,600					
1,500					
1,400					
1,300					
1,200					

MILES
2   4   6   7.8

#2, Bar-O Pasture Trail, just on this side of West Verde Creek. Turn left here. West Verde Creek is on your right and the hills of Twin Peaks are to the left. Ahead, Trail #2B leaves right—keep forward to meet Trail #2A, Creek Bottom Trail, at 0.5 miles. Turn right here, immediately stepping over the streambed of West Verde Creek. Begin cruising thick woods bordering the park boundary fence. At just over a mile, a boundary fence gate leads right to a private equestrian lodge. Veer left here, looking for a quick right turn onto a singletrack path. Do not stay forward on the wide roadbed—you will end at the closed park road. The singletrack path, the correct trail, goes over a small berm and beside an old pond bed to the right before entering dense and appealing woods.

Ahead, the woods open a bit—songbirds accompany the deep green hue of the juniper, contrasting with the brown grass at your feet and the brilliant blue Texas sky overhead. At nearly 2 miles, in a live oak thicket, pick up Trail #3, Hermit's Trace. Begin to climb and remember to look back for good views to the south and west. Climb over a couple of deep washes to reach a trail junction at about 2.5 miles. Turn right here, picking up Trail #3A, Good Luck Trail. This is named for the luck you'll need in surmounting its steep ups and downs. Immediately start your first ascent. Gravity will prove that you really are in Texas Hill Country. The junipers offer enough space between them to allow views all around and the knowledge that you are heading into a bowl encircled by ridges.

At nearly 3 miles, Trail #3B (with no alternative name) leaves to the left. Keep going forward, keep climbing, and then dip into a densely wooded wash. Begin a lung-buster climb on a rocky trail to top out on a ridge. Gather yourself and then begin an equally steep descent to meet a rock wash at mile 3.4. Just ahead, Trail #3B comes in from the left; stay right here to meet Trail #3, Hermit's Trace. Hermit's Trace is a doubletrack path. This is an important junction. To your right, 0.3 miles away, in the uppermost reaches of West Verde Creek Valley, is the Hermit's Shack Camp Area for equestrians and backpackers. Turn left here, passing the Butterfly Springs Camp Area on your right, which is for backpackers only. Cross West Verde Creek.

Keep down the valley, working around a wide-open wash that used to be spanned by a bridge. You can still see the soil abutment of the bridge. Watch for an old wooden shack on your right beyond the abutment. At 4.2 miles, look right for the singletrack Cougar Canyon Trail, Trail #4. Take the Cougar Canyon Trail across the bed of West Verde Creek, where skeletal oaks were probably killed in a fire from times past. The Panther Canyon draw is to your left. At 4.5 miles, Trail #4A, the Cougar Canyon Overlook Trail, leaves right. This dead-end path heads a half mile to the hill above, as well as a far-reaching vista (total hike mileage does not include this side trip).

The Cougar Canyon Trail crosses Cougar Canyon on an old pond dam before dipping to a small wash and ascending the ridge dead ahead. Top out on the ridge, where Trail #4B (with no other name) leaves to the right. You will likely notice the view ahead more than the trail leaving right. Here the West

Verde Valley stretches far in the distance, far to the east. Begin working down the valley in broken juniper woodland, passing an old tin shack in the next wash, which is wooded with live oak. Come along a fence line. Ahead you can see the park group lodge.

At 5.8 miles pass through a gate. Trail #4 goes both ways. Turn right here and soon come to a boarded house on your left. At the house Trail #4B goes right. Stay left on Hermit's Trace and cross the dam of an old pond. Reach another trail junction in moist woods at 6.3 miles. Turn left here onto Trail #5, Twin Peaks Trail. Dip through shady oaks and other hardwoods before briefly opening into juniper. Return to lush woods with many a tall tree along a flat by West Verde Creek. Sycamores line the banks of the streambed. Shortly you'll reach the park road, which is closed to private vehicular traffic, near a culvert. Turn right here and walk a short distance before veering left onto Trail #2, Bar-O Pasture Trail. The grass and soil footing and the wide-open valley bottom contrast greatly with the rocky hills through which you've been traveling.

Keep in grassland through the heart of the valley. At 7.3 miles, intersect Trail #2A, Creek Bottom Trail. This completes the loop portion of the trek. Keep forward on Trail #2, backtracking to Trail #6, and return to the trailhead.

NEARBY ACTIVITIES

Hill Country State Natural Area offers walk-in tent camping, backpacking, bicycling, horseback riding, and fishing.

KERRVILLE-SCHREINER PARK LOOP

58

IN BRIEF

This loop hike encompasses several trails at this park just outside the city of Kerrville. Ramble through juniper woods, topping out at a high point where you can overlook the Guadalupe River Valley below. Circle back off the hilltop to complete the loop. The many different trails here offer other loop combinations for hikers and mountain bikers.

DESCRIPTION

The trails here at Kerrville-Schreiner Park, once a Texas state park but now transferred to the city of Kerrville, are color coded. You will be traveling a series of these paths to make a loop. A park map is a definite help in making this route, but it is not so complicated as this narrative implies when you are in the field with map in hand. So don't get so caught up in staying on the correct trail that you miss all the scenery!

Leave Trailhead #3 and immediately enter a shady juniper forest on the Yellow Trail. Plastic posts indicating the trail have been placed at trail intersections. A color-coded

----

Directions

From San Antonio head north on I-10 to Exit 508, TX 16. Take TX 16 south and travel 0.3 miles to east Loop Road 534. Turn left on Loop Road 534. Keep forward on Loop 534, crossing the Guadalupe River, and reach TX 173 at 4.3 miles. Turn left on TX 173, and immediately turn right to enter Kerrville-Schreiner Park. From the park entrance, turn left on Park Road 19 and travel 0.4 miles to an intersection. Turn left again, heading toward the camping area and the trailhead, Trailhead #3, will be on your left after 0.4 miles. The trailhead is just beyond the right turn into the park group shelter.

KEY AT-A-GLANCE INFORMATION

LENGTH: 3.5 miles

CONFIGURATION: Loop

DIFFICULTY: Moderate

SCENERY: Hill Country woods

EXPOSURE: Mostly open

TRAFFIC: Moderate

TRAIL SURFACE: Gravel, rock, dirt

HIKING TIME: 2.5 hours

DRIVING DISTANCE: 66 miles from the Alamo

ACCESS: Daily, 8 a.m.–10 p.m.; $4 day-use fee/person over age 13; $2 day-use fee/senior; $1 day-use fee/child

WHEELCHAIR ACCESS: No

MAPS: kerrville.org

FACILITIES: Water, restrooms at nearby campground

CONTACT INFORMATION: (830) 257-5392; kerrville.org

GPS TRAILHEAD COORDINATES

LATITUDE: 30° 00' 09.17"
LONGITUDE: 99° 12' 83.06"

58 Kerrville–Schreiner Park Loop

N | 0 — 0.15 — 0.3 mile

To 10

173

534

Bandera Highway

Memorial Pkwy.

park headquarters

maintenance building

toll booth

173

Park Road 19

Deer Field Campground

Mountain View Campground

Fawn Hide-a-Way Campground

Highpoint Campground

group dining hall

Fox Run Campground

cabin

KERRVILLE–SCHREINER PARK

Y Yellow Trail
B Blue Trail
R Red Trail
O Orange Trail
G Green Trail

band with an accompanying arrow is atop the plastic post. Occasional oaks and grass vary the woodland. At 0.1 mile the pea-gravel portion of the path, an all-access trail, splits left and goes to an overlook beyond the park boundary. Keep forward on the Yellow Trail, coming alongside a rock shelf to the left. The trail opens to a fence line marking the park border. Here you can enjoy views of the hills, cattle country, and creeping suburbanization.

The forest opens. Look for narrow deer paths crisscrossing the trail. At almost 1 mile, veer left onto the Blue Trail, staying with it for nearly 0.5 miles, and pick up the Orange Trail. Stay left on a narrower path, ascending to reach another junction at almost 1.5 miles. Stay left again as the Orange Trail splits. Begin to climb steadily on a rooty track, and gain the hilltop just below a water tower. Here you can look through the juniper trees onto the Guadalupe Valley below.

The Guadalupe River flowing through the Hill Country originally attracted Native Americans, who lived in the area off and on for 10,000 years; white settlers came in the early 1800s. The town of Kerrville was perched on a bluff near the river. Originally a shingle maker's camp named Brownsborough, it became Kerrville in the 1850s. But it wasn't until a pair of German settlers built a mill here that the town began to grow. This growth spawned Charles A. Schreiner's multifaceted businesses, which in turn spurred the further growth of Kerrville. Schreiner shares the name of the park near the town he helped develop.

Descend along the fence line marking the park boundary, making an acute right turn, heading toward the interior of the park and more trail junctions. The path is mostly shady here. The Orange Trail splits again—stay left, keeping downhill. The country opens up and grasses become more common. Now intersect the Green Trail at just over 2 miles. Stay right here, dipping through a small wash. The Green Trail goes both ways at the next junction—stay right. All these junctions are a pain, but this loop is attempting to cover the most scenic ground and still make sense.

Intersect the Blue Trail at 2.3 miles. Turn left here and follow it a short distance before it splits. Turn right, leaving the roadbed and joining a rocky track. Ahead at 2.7 miles is the final intersection. It may seem oddly familiar, and it is. Turn left here, rejoining the Yellow Trail to backtrack to the trailhead, perhaps wishing that you had brought a global positioning system.

NEARBY ACTIVITIES

Kerrville-Schreiner Park has fishing on the Guadalupe River, as well as camping, hiking, and mountain biking.

59 PANTHER CANYON TRAIL

KEY AT-A-GLANCE INFORMATION

LENGTH: 1.6 miles

CONFIGURATION: Out-and-back

DIFFICULTY: Moderate

SCENERY: Wooded canyon

EXPOSURE: Mostly shady

TRAFFIC: Moderate, busy on warm-weather weekends

TRAIL SURFACE: Rocks, dirt

HIKING TIME: 1 hour

DRIVING DISTANCE: 33 miles from the Alamo

ACCESS: Daily, 6 a.m.–midnight; no fees or permits (but $10 picnic-table fee)

WHEELCHAIR ACCESS: No

MAPS: nbtexas.org/index .aspx?nid=1184

FACILITIES: Restrooms, water fountains at park

CONTACT INFORMATION: (830) 221-4350; tx-newbraunfels.civicplus .com/index.aspx?NID=156

GPS TRAILHEAD COORDINATES

LATITUDE: 29° 71' 04.17"
LONGITUDE: 98° 13' 53.89"

IN BRIEF

This is a surprisingly scenic hike up a lush canyon in Landa Park, a New Braunfels city park that is worth visiting in its own right. In addition to enjoying the scenery, you can enhance your knowledge of the canyon's flora and fauna with interpretive information available at the park office. Deer are often spotted in the depths of the canyon. Give yourself plenty of time to enjoy not only the trail but the rest of Landa Park as well.

DESCRIPTION

The trail begins at Comal Springs, the headwaters of the Comal River, around which Landa Park is centered. However, Panther Canyon is dry, heavy rains excepted. Along the way you will crisscross the wet-weather streambed beneath rich woodland covering the canyon floor and hills. Sheer rock bluffs add a scenic touch to the walk. Landa Park also has a paved walking and jogging trail that winds through the park. Stop by the park office to pick up the interpretive guide for the

----

Directions

From Exit 187 on I-35 in New Braunfels, take Seguin Avenue west, going around the town square. At 1.4 miles, veer left onto Landa Street from Seguin Avenue. Follow Landa Street to enter Landa Park. Turn right into Landa Park and keep forward on Landa Park Drive, crossing the Comal River a total of three times (the first crossing is just after you enter the park). After the third crossing and a total of 0.6 miles, look right for the parking area beside a spring wading pool. Comal Springs is just across the street from the parking area. The Panther Canyon Trail begins just beyond the springhead.

Hairy Cave ▲

Comal Springs

LANDA PARK

park office

Comal River

Ohio Street

California Street

Landa Street

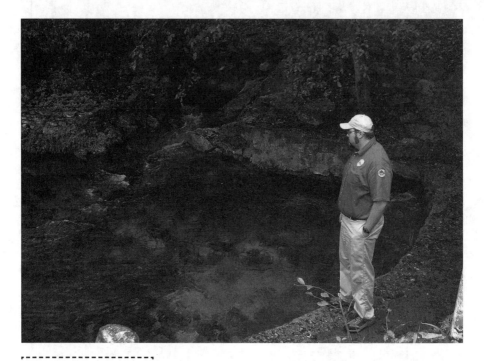

Checking out Comal Springs

Panther Canyon Trail. Numbered posts along the trail correspond with the interpretive literature.

Landa Park and Comal Springs have an interesting history. Located along
the Balcones Fault, the springs, heralded as the biggest springs in Texas and the
Southwest, issue forth from the Edwards Aquifer. The level land of the park area
was a popular camping spot for Texas's Native Americans. Many artifacts and
burial sites have been found around the springs. A Spanish mission was built here
in 1756. Later, German settlers came to the area, naming the community New
Braunfels. William H. Merriweather bought the Comal Springs tract in 1847,
building a cotton gin and gristmill. Joseph Landa later purchased it. In the late
1800s, the area known as Landa's Pasture became a popular picnicking place.
Comal Springs' reputation as a tourist destination grew, attracting a railroad line
and hotel. Excursion rails ran from San Antonio and Austin, carrying passengers
to visit and bathe in the springs.

The Landa property was sold, and the tract suffered during the Great Depression and was eventually closed as a park. The closure prompted the city of New
Braunfels to purchase the property in 1936. Since then, the park has been
expanded with additional purchases and development, becoming the destination
it is today.

The Panther Canyon area was one of the later purchases forming the modern
Landa Park. Stop and check out Comal Springs at the trailhead. The water is clear,

cool, and clean as it busts directly out of a limestone wall. The spring harbors the endangered fountain darter, a small fish. Pass the springs and enter the surprisingly narrow, deep, and natural Panther Canyon, which contrasts greatly with the balance of the wide-open, manicured park. Immediately cross the first wash. Overhead is a wealth of trees, including live oak, elm, buckeye, and mountain laurel.

At a bench, look across the canyon for a small cave, really more of a narrow, tunnel-like opening. This is an old spring mouth, now dry, known as Hairy Cave. During the summer, the cave is so thick with granddaddy longlegs that the inside appears to be hairy! Try to keep quiet as you ascend the canyon. Deer are present here—you may see one, especially if you're here in the morning and evening.

Keep crisscrossing back and forth over a rocky streambed. Watch for sheer, moss-covered walls. The canyon opens up and widens in places. Here the hardwoods grow over a pretty grassy understory. The trail curves with the canyon, continuing to ascend. Side washes come in occasionally. At nearly a mile, reach the park boundary near a private residence to your left. This is a good turnaround spot. However, an informal path continues up the canyon to Ohio Street and New Braunfels High School.

NEARBY ACTIVITIES

Landa Park is a fun destination. Here you can not only hike but also swim in a spring-fed pool or an Olympic-size conventional pool, picnic, ride a mini-train, and fish. Other pastimes include golf, miniature golf, and tennis. The park also has a concrete walking and jogging trail. The nearby Guadalupe River has tubing in summer.

60   TWIN PEAKS TRAIL

KEY AT-A-GLANCE INFORMATION

LENGTH: 3 miles

CONFIGURATION: Loop

DIFFICULTY: Moderate

SCENERY: Typical Hill Country vegetation ranging from mountain cedar to Spanish dagger (yucca)

EXPOSURE: Open

TRAFFIC: Moderate–heavy

TRAIL SURFACE: Dirt and rock, some loose gravel

HIKING TIME: 1.5 hours

DRIVING DISTANCE: 52 miles from the Alamo

ACCESS: Daily, 8 a.m.–10 p.m.; closed during public hunts; $6 day-use fee/person over age 13

WHEELCHAIR ACCESS: No

MAPS: tpwd.state.tx.us/ publications

FACILITIES: Untreated water, privy at park headquarters

CONTACT INFORMATION: (830) 796-4413; tpwd.state.tx.us/spdest/ findadest/parks/hill_country

GPS TRAILHEAD COORDINATES

LATITUDE: 29° 62' 73.06"
LONGITUDE: 99° 17' 80.56"

IN BRIEF

This rugged hike up a central Texas hill will take you to one of the best views around for miles; it is followed up with a stroll down to the valley you were viewing from the peak.

DESCRIPTION

Hill Country State Natural Area is as rugged as a park can get and still attract visitors. A haven for horse lovers, mountain bikers, and hikers alike, this park was designed solely for their use. Deeded to the Texas Parks and Wildlife Department under conditions that it is kept as wild and natural as possible, this area has had little done in the way of improvements. No water or electricity is available in the park, so unless campers bring a generator, they are limited to roughing it. Even with such conditions, campers should make reservations, as only 10 campsites are in the park.

The only other improvements made here are the marked trails (more than 40 miles) and the horse stables in both the day-use and campsite areas. Hikers, riders, and bikers alike are allowed to use all the trails in the park, and rules of the road have been established to ensure peaceful cohabitation. While on the trails, bikers yield to hikers and horses, and hikers yield to horses. This is to keep horses from getting

----

Directions ⟶

From San Antonio take TX 16 to Bandera. In Bandera, turn left on TX 173 south, following it for one mile to FR 1077. Turn right onto FR 1077 and follow it for 10 miles to the park, where the road turns to dirt. Turn right into the park, crossing West Verde Creek, and then turn right into the parking area near the park headquarters. A ranger will point you to the trailhead parking area.

spooked and hurting themselves or others. These rules are enforced with citations by the rangers, who are also law-enforcement officers. They will also cite visitors for straying off the trails. Do not go cross-country during your hikes here.

The park office is a simple portable building with a bulletin board. When you're checking in, the rangers will be happy to show various trail highlights on the map, as well as to explain the symbols used to denote hazardous areas. Scenic areas are also marked, and the map is much more detailed than most state park maps. This park is for trailblazers. The trailhead is located in the camping areas west of the office. Park there and head to the trailhead between campsites 214 and 215, located about 0.1 mile from the parking spaces. Do not park in the campsites.

Trails in the park are numbered and marked with signs at intersections and points along the trails. Follow the trail from the campsites into the brush toward two obvious hills that almost appear to be connected. The dirt trail is narrow at this point, and it gradually climbs from the camping area. You'll reach a T-intersection 0.3 miles into the trail. Continue to the left to make your way to the two hills. From here the view already gets breathtaking. To your left you can see a good deal of the park, as you've climbed more than 100 feet above the parking area.

The trail intersects Trail 6 just 0.5 miles from the trailhead. You will turn here later. For now, remain on the trail you're on, which will fork 0.1 mile from the intersection. Continue left toward the peak and the view that awaits there. From here the trail becomes loose gravel and can be tricky. A section of trail is fashioned into crude steps using telephone-type poles and gravel. Don't let this slight improvement cause you to let your guard down. Watch your step. This is one of the areas on the map marked as treacherous. The peak is another 0.2 miles up the trail. From an elevation of 1,886 feet, look east to see the camping area you just hiked through. From the rest of the peak you can view the rolling hills and cedars that make up this area of Texas. You should also be able to see horseback riders along the many trails visible from here. You can easily imagine yourself in the Texas of 150 years ago.

As you come back down the hill the way you came, you'll return to the intersection with Trail 6. Take this fork to the right and meander through the valley you were just appreciating. The narrow trail wanders through cedar, live oak, and mesquite that are never really high enough to provide adequate shade. Attentive hikers have a good chance to catch sight of deer walking along the trail, stopping to browse on the numerous plants and herbs.

The trail continues for 0.8 miles, at which point it intersects Trail 1. Turn left onto this new trail that will lead you back to your vehicle. The path here is wide enough for vehicular traffic (which is not allowed) and shows obvious signs of use by both bikers and horseback riders. The trail almost sets a leisurely pace for you on the wide path, reminiscent of an old country road. It narrows to single-hiker width a half mile from the last intersection but quickly widens again afterward.

At 2.7 miles into your hike, you'll reach another fork that leads off Trail 5A. Stay on your present course, which will emerge in the campground 0.2 miles from the fork between campsites 215 and 216. Turn right here and head back to your car for fresh water before tackling one of the park's many other trails.

APPENDIXES
AND INDEX

APPENDIX A:

HIKING STORES

AUSTIN

REI
rei.com
9901 North Capital of Texas
  Highway, Suite 200
(512) 343-5550

601 North Lamar Boulevard
(512) 482-3357

WHOLE EARTH PROVISION COMPANY
wholeearthprovision.com
1014 North Lamar Boulevard
(512) 476-1414

4477 South Lamar Boulevard,
  Suite 200
(512) 899-0992

SAN ANTONIO

NATIONAL OUTDOORS
5600 Bandera Road
(210) 680-3322

6900 San Pedro Avenue
(210) 979-8111

SPORTS AUTHORITY
sportsauthority.com
125 Northwest Loop 410, Suite 140
(210) 341-1244

WHOLE EARTH PROVISION COMPANY
wholeearthprovision.com
255 East Basse Road, Suite 510
(210) 829-8888

APPENDIX B:

PLACES TO BUY MAPS

AUSTIN

MAPSCO MAP & TRAVEL CENTER
mapsco.com
6406 North IH-35, Suite 1301
(888) 674-6277
(512) 302-9036

WHOLE EARTH PROVISION COMPANY
wholeearthprovision.com
1014 North Lamar Boulevard
(512) 476-1414

4477 South Lamar Boulevard,
   Suite 200
(512) 899-0992

SAN ANTONIO

MAPSCO MAP & TRAVEL CENTER
mapsco.com
610 West Sunset Road
(800) 798-2112
(210) 829-7629

WHOLE EARTH PROVISION COMPANY
wholeearthprovision.com
255 East Basse Road, Suite 510
(210) 829-8888

APPENDIX C:
HIKING CLUBS

ALAMO GROUP OF THE SIERRA CLUB
texas.sierraclub.org/alamo
P.O. Box 6443
San Antonio, TX 78209

AUSTIN HIKING GROUP
meetup.com/austin-hikers

AUSTIN REGIONAL GROUP OF THE SIERRA CLUB
texas.sierraclub.org/austin
P.O. Box 4581
Austin, TX 78765-5392

CENTRAL TEXAS TRAIL TAMERS
trailtamers.org
P.O. Box 12045
Austin, TX 78711-2045
(512) 394-9998

COLORADO RIVER WALKERS
coloradoriverwalkers.org
(512) 281-0741

HILL COUNTRY OUTDOORS
hillcountryoutdoors.com
P.O. Box 684732
Austin, TX 78768-4732
(512) 383-1191

SAN ANTONIO HIKING & OUTDOORS GROUP
meetup.com/saoutdoors

INDEX